National Library of Australia Cataloguing-in-Publication entry

Author: Phillips, Karen.

Title: Mom please help : anorexia-bulimia, positive
               energy reatment./Karen Phillips, Dr. Irina
               Webster; editor, William Webster BA.

ISBN: 9780646492780 (pbk.)

Notes: Bibliography.

Subjects: Anorexia nervosa—Treatment.
               Bulimia—Treatment.
               Eating disorders.

Other Authors/Contributors:
               Webster, Irina Dr.
               Webster, William.

Dewey Number: 616.8526

ANOREXIA & BULIMIA
'Positive Energy Treatment'

— COINED BY **Dr. Irina Webster**

Mom, Please Help

KAREN PHILLIPS

Disclaimer

This book intends to educate and teach people about how they can use Neuroplasticity to overcome their eating disorders. The reader takes all responsibility for her/his use of the material written in the book. The result of the treatment can vary, depending on how people use it.

The views and advice expressed in this book are not intended to be a substitute for conventional medical services. If you have any concerns regarding your (or your loved one's) condition, see physician of choice.

ISBN 978-0-646-49278-0

Dedication

I dedicate this book to all mothers, fathers, grandmothers, grand-fathers, sisters, brothers, spouses, friends, and relatives of those who happen to be affected by eating disorders—and to all those who have passed on because of it.

I dedicate this book to those who have the courage, love, and the heart to fight these insidious disorders and who have the courage to help their loved ones recover.

Some names in this book have been changed to protect their identity and confidentiality. All of the symptoms and the treat-ment methods are portrayed as they actually occurred.

Acknowledgements

This book could not have been written without the help, inspiration, and support of Dr. Irina Webster, MD and her husband William Webster, BA. I used the knowledge and encouragement they've shared with me from the first time I met them—and until now. They gave me insight to my actions, and guidance when I had to cope with the illness of my daughter in the late stages of recovery.

They were the first people who taught me about the amazing ability of the brain to change itself: Neuroplasticity.

They were the first to teach me that the best way to utilize the power of Neuroplasticity is to be in a state of Mindful Awareness. I believe this is the only way to create positive changes in the brain and transform your self to become the best you can be.

I want to thank Norman Dodge, MD, whose "The Brain that Changes Itself" made me see the brain and mind from a different perspective and pointed me in the right direction regarding the management of my daughter's eating disorder.

I am grateful to Bruce Lipton, PhD for his insight and research in cellular biology. He is the person who showed that our beliefs, true or false, positive or negative, affect genetic activity and can actually alter our genetic code. His discovery completely transformed my mind as a mother who was helping her anorexic daughter recover, and made me question the traditional approach to eating disorders.

Also, I want to thank Jeffrey M. Schwartz, MD, who successfully proved that Neuroplasticity methods can cure OCD (obsessive-compulsive disorders). I was really excited to read about this as I had a long-standing view that an eating disorder was a form of OCD (but in connection to food and weight). His methods inspired me to continue to work with my daughter and help her fully recover from her anorexia-bulimia.

I needed a lot of help, knowledge, information, and experience from others to write this book about my efforts and discoveries. I would like to thank everyone who has provided this service and assistance to me.

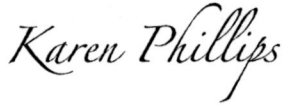

Contents

INTRODUCTION

Why I Wrote
Mom, Please Help

*I*f you have ordered this book from my website, www.
mom-please-help.com, then you have probably read the
story of how I was able to help my daughter Amy to recover from a severe eating disorder.

I did not discover the methods I describe in this book from
doctors, psychiatrists or psychologists. I came upon them after
reading a lot of books, attending many seminars, and talking to
many sufferers and helpers. We call this method "Positive Energy Treatment."

Not all of my studies or information I learned was about eating disorders. Some were about how to change your emotions
and feelings and get in touch with your subconscious mind. I

talked and listened to famous people like Dr. Deepak Chopra, Anthony Robbins, John Gray, and Gregg Jacobs, Ph.D., because they all talk about changing your emotional state, and how important this is in leading a healthy psychological life.

From talking to psychologists and doctors, I learned that an eating disorder is a disease of feelings and emotions. How to change these feelings and emotions permanently was something they did not know, as it was outside their training.

Doctors just prescribed Amy some drugs (antidepressants and anti-anxiety medication) and sent her for counseling. Amy did not like the drugs because they made her even sicker, so she did not take them.

Psychologists told me to be patient and gave me some hints on how to cope, but they did not tell me exactly how to change Amy's feelings, thoughts, and emotions.

That is why I went to see Dr. Deepak Chopra and Anthony Robbins and paid big money to attend. What they taught me really made a lot of sense and helped me format my plan to help Amy.

I read a lot about the statistics of eating disorders and they shocked me.

Research suggests that about one percent (1%) of female adolescents have anorexia. The latest figures from the USA suggest that it could be higher than 8% of the population. This means that about one out of every one hundred young women between ten and twenty are starving themselves, sometimes to death! And for the general population this is a staggering eight out of every one hundred.

Research suggests that about four percent (4%), or four out of one hundred, college-aged women have bulimia. About 50% of people who have been anorexic develop bulimia or bulimic patterns.

Because people with bulimia are secretive, it is difficult to know how many older people are affected. Bulimia is rare in young children.

Dieting teens: More than half of teenaged girls are, or think they should be, on diets. They want to lose all or some of the forty pounds that females naturally gain between 8 and 14 years of age. About three percent of these teens go too far, becoming anorexic or bulimic.

I was very successful in my attempts in treating my daughter and her eating disorder using my own approach (nobody told me to do exactly what I did). Because of this I decided to write this book to share all my knowledge with other people and to help them cure their eating problems.

But now I have the added advantage of having the input of a doctor who was a sufferer herself. She did not use the normal stuff she was taught as a doctor to cure herself, because she tried that and it did not work. So like me, she formulated a new approach outside traditional methods, and came up with a treatment program similar to mine.

This is what you will learn in this book.

Disclaimer

The statements in this book have not been evaluated by the Food and Drug Administration. The products and information mentioned in this book are not intended to diagnose, treat, cure, or prevent any disease. Information and statements made are for education purposes and are not intended to replace the advice of your doctor.

The views and advice expressed in this book are not intended to be a substitute for conventional medical services. If you have a severe medical condition, see your physician of choice.

> *"One cannot think well, love well, sleep well, if one has not dined well."*
>
> ~ Virginia Woolf

CHAPTER 1

Our Story: How It All Began

My name is Karen Phillips and this is the story of my daughter Amy, who suffered from—and survived—anorexia and bulimia. I thank God everyday for answering my prayers for her recovery.

Well I guess it was 11 years ago when I started to notice something was not right with Amy. She had just turned 13 when I caught her always looking at herself in the mirror. She would ask me if I thought she had put on weight. I told her of course she hadn't—she always looked just right for her age.

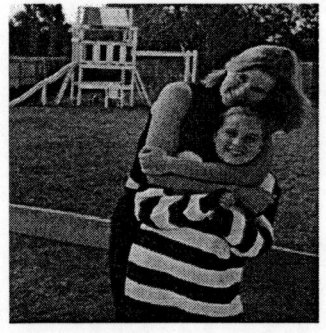

Here we were (left) just a year before she developed her first symptoms of the eating disorder. As you can see, she looked happy and was a nice-looking young girl.

You know, I never even thought anything was wrong! I took it as just "being a teenager" thing, and really thought no more about it. I remember myself in those teenage years, worrying about my looks and going on diets and other similar, trivial stuff. It was what a lot of my friends did, too.

I didn't even pick up on the fact that Amy would just play with her food at the dinner table and just move everything around her plate, eating very little. Of course I would ask her why she didn't eat her food, but she would just say that she had a lot to eat at school or at a friend's place or some other excuse¬—and I would fall for it each time.

Now, in hindsight, I feel really guilty, as a mom, for not being more aware of things at that time, and I go through the "if only I had noticed back then, I maybe could have done something" sentiment each time. But I didn't notice anything peculiar, and before I knew it, 10 years of living hell was about to begin.

Amy had always been a beautiful, intelligent girl—always thinking of other people, always nice and kind. When she was 8, she would always do things for her grandmother (who had come to live with us). She always asked if she needed help cleaning, or if she could do anything for her. She always volunteered to take Gran's dinner to her and bring back the dirty dishes; nothing was too much for her.

Amy was 12 when her grandmother passed away. We thought she would be really upset, but she seemed to handle it better than anyone. Even her younger brother Ben seemed more upset. We put it down to the fact that Gran had been sick for over 6 months and we had explained to her that Gran would not live that much longer. Even at the funeral, Amy did not cry; she seemed to be in full control. But then again, I was too upset about losing my Mom that I did not really pay attention.

My God! What an idiot I was back then. How could I have missed all the little signals that Amy was sending me? Why didn't I see the warning signs? They were all there to be seen, but I didn't notice a thing. How could I have been so stupid?

I think what really sent Amy on the trip that nearly cost her life was a major disappointment that happened when she was 13. Amy loved to dance, and she was good at it. She had a real passion for dancing. She always said that she wanted to be a dancer when she grew up, and if any dancing came on TV, she would not miss it. Even if there was a family outing or a birthday party, if dancing was on TV, she would refuse to go until the show is done.

I have to tell you, at this point, Amy was not a typical little 13-year-old. She was quite developed for her age, with breasts and more of a mature shape to her body. She was more like a

16-year-old. Most of her friends were still waiting to develop breasts and were still thin little girls with no shape. I didn't know it then, but Amy was teased about her body by some of the girls at school. They would call her fat and tell her she had a big bottom. Of course, this was not true. Amy was just more developed, but she was starting to think she was really fat.

The events of 18th of November 1994, I believe, were the catalysts for the 10 years of hell. It was the auditions for the Christmas extravaganza. Amy had been practicing for months to get into the school dance troupe and she wanted so badly to get the lead dance role. Two days before the auditions, she got ill. By the time her dance trials came, she was not in good health. She failed to get the lead role; in fact she danced so badly she did not even make the team. When she was leaving the stage, I heard one of the successful girls say, "I told you you're too fat."

Amy was inconsolable. She screamed and yelled and cried and cried. I tried to console her by saying that there was always next year and it was not her fault that she was sick, but nothing could comfort her. "I had tried so hard," she wailed. "Why was I not picked? Mom, I wanted to be in the show. Why did I not get in? I am too fat; they didn't pick me because I am too fat."

Amy just sobbed and sobbed all night in her room and there was nothing I could do, absolutely nothing. I remember saying to my husband John that she will cry herself out and in a couple of days, she would be that lovable girl we know. How wrong this statement turned out to be.

I have heard anorexia described by another sufferer as being "like getting on an escalator that you can't get off." It just keeps going and you don't even know how you got on in the first place. All you know is the floor has changed. You think you are in control at first, but then it takes control of you and there is nothing you can do about it. This is basically what happened to Amy; I believe she got on the escalator the night of the auditions looking for something she could control, but only found the devil.

Amy seemed to recover a bit after a few weeks but became more aloof and withdrawn. To us, she seemed to be eating okay, and we thought she was getting over her disappointments. She even wanted to go see the show, as some of her friends were going. But when it came to the night of the show, she said she had a headache and stayed in her room. Of course this was also another signal that all was not well with Amy.

One of the major indicators of an eating disorder is the sufferer becomes more and more withdrawn. But it is so subtle; it is extremely hard for someone on the outside to notice.

Over the next 12 months, Amy seemed to be doing well in school. Her grades were up and she was near the top of her class. But she had completely given up on her dancing, saying that she wanted to concentrate on her schoolwork. Amy had always liked going to school even when she was little. In fact, she couldn't wait to get back to school during the term breaks, always looking forward to the new school year. So when she told us she wanted to do better at school, we simply believed her. After all, her grades reflected all the effort she was putting in. We didn't realize that, in reality, she was withdrawing further and further into herself.

She wasn't eating much, and soon started to look thin and scrawny. I never noticed her weight loss as it was winter, and she wore bulky clothing that covered her up. It was only well into spring, when she started to wear slimmer-fitting clothes, that I really saw the extent of the problem.

I started to worry about this, but when I'd approach her, she would tell me she was just on a diet. She told me not to bother her. It was at this time that the alarm bells started to go off in my head; *she was starting to look really emaciated.* To me she looked like one of those photos you see of people in the concentration camps—all skin and bones, hair lank and without luster. My God, I started to think, what is going on here?

It was time for us to confront Amy to see what in the world was happening. We decided to wait until Ben, her brother, was not home, as we wanted to have a good talk with Amy. We reckoned it would be a more relaxed atmosphere if he was not there. But what transpired was anything but relaxed…

Amy just did not want to talk. She exploded—swearing and cursing at us, telling us that it was her life, and if she wanted to diet she would. I said to her that she had no fat to lose. She was just skin and bones. She pointed to her shoulders, asked me if I was blind and to look at "all the fat" on her shoulder. I tried to point out that it was the bone in her arm, not fat. She yelled and screamed, called me an idiot and said that she just wanted us to leave her alone. Then she slammed the door in our face.

I was in absolute shock. Tears were streaming down my face. What had just happened? I couldn't believe what I was hearing. I would learn later on that this reaction is common among anorexia sufferers and is called "broken eye syndrome."

John tried to open the door but it was locked. He yelled for Amy to open the door; he wanted answers right then. All we got back was a tirade of abuse. He banged on the door but Amy just got worse and worse, yelling and screaming. We heard things being thrown and smashed, and Amy telling us to go away and let her be.

I was distraught. Oh my God! What was going on? I couldn't understand. I thought I was a good mother. I was just totally unprepared for this. I was in a state of denial. How could this be? This was not the beautiful little girl I knew; this was some kind of monster that has come into my life.

I called my doctor to talk to him; I needed answers. He suggested that I come and see him and bring Amy if it was possible, so I made an appointment for the next day. When Amy calmed down, I asked her if she wanted to go with me. She refused, asking why would she want to go to see a doctor when there was nothing wrong with her. I wanted to say something but the events of that morning stopped me; I did not want a repeat performance until I at least knew what it is I was dealing with.

I attended the appointment with Dr. Thomson and explained what had happened. He asked me a number of questions about Amy and then told me he was sure that she had an eating disorder and it was probably anorexia.

Well, I nearly fell of my chair! I just could not understand how in the world this had happened to Amy. I knew absolutely nothing about anorexia, except what I had read about movie stars who supposedly had all these kinds of problems through the stress of keeping thin for their careers. But Amy was only a little girl. *She was my little girl.* She didn't have these kinds of pressures. How could she have anorexia?

Dr. Thomson told me what he could and recommended we get Amy to see a counselor as soon as possible. He told me that people die because of anorexia and it is a psychological problem, not an eating one. He explained that the eating is a symptom of a bigger problem and we had to get to the bottom of the problem to fix it. There was nothing he could prescribe, getting her to a counselor was her only chance—or she could die.

I sat there completely dumbfounded; my little girl could die. I didn't know what to say. My heart was in my mouth, tears were flowing down my face, and I was shaking as all color drained from my face. I could see the concern in the doctor's eyes and he advised me to just relax for a moment.

She was only 14; how could she die? I went to see the doctor thinking he would tell me it was just a normal teenage thing and not to worry, that she would grow out of it. I didn't expect to be told that my baby could die.

That was it. Amy was going to see a counselor even if I had to drag her screaming and yelling every inch of the way. I was resolute; there was no way she was going to die. Not if I had anything to do with it. I would go home and force-feed her if I had to. I was not going to sit back and watch her die. At the time, I was thinking like any mother would given the situation. I did not know then how complicated this disease really is, but I was about to find that out the hard way.

We did get Amy to go and see a counselor—and a very good one—for this kind of problem. For the next 2 years we battled Amy's devils and we thought we were starting to get on top of things. It was during these sessions that we found out that Amy had taken the death of her grandmother extremely badly and had bottled up all the emotions. Also, missing out on the dance performance on top of all the bad emotions was a major turning point in Amy's life. To us it was a molehill; to Amy it was Mount Everest.

During the next 2 years, I read and studied everything I could find on anorexia. It was during this time that I started to think about the methods I would later put into action, and which ones would change everything.

Amy seemed to be hanging in there and, although she did not start to have any significant weight gain, she did improve —actually, "seemed to improve" may be a better way of saying it.

After about 15 months, Amy all of a sudden started to eat more. We were overjoyed. She would even eat more than her brother sometimes, and he was a big eater. We thought we were overcoming the problem and even though she did not put on weight, we were not that concerned. We simply thought that after nearly 4 years of virtual starvation, it would take the body a little while to revert to a normal metabolism.

We never even noticed that Amy had started to binge eat and then purge herself, not only after dinner, but after every meal. I was well aware that this could happen and I did keep an eye out, but Amy was very sneaky. She would go to the bathroom downstairs, in the pool area, where she knew no one would go. Of course we didn't find out until it was too late.

It was August 24th 1999, and we had to go away for 3 weeks on business. We received a phone call from my sister Betty who was looking after the house and kids. She said that Amy had collapsed at home and was in the hospital. We were told that things were not looking good, and that we had better get back soon.

I totally panicked. I had promised myself that no way was I going to let Amy die and now there was a strong possibility that it just may happen.

The recriminations started to come thick and fast in my head. Why did I go away? Why didn't I see what was happening? It was all my fault. I was a bad mother! I was worried sick…

We got to the hospital 12 hours later, catching the first plane out that we could get. Amy was on a drip and looked very ill. My heart fell. I was so worried; this was the worst I have ever seen Amy look, and I feared I was going to lose her. Amy was in and out of consciousness. I just sat there and prayed to God that he let her live.

The doctors told me her potassium level was 1.9, which is very low—low enough that her heart could stop beating. This was the worst time in my life. Sitting there thinking you are about to lose a child is the most emotionally traumatic thing you can go through, and to this day my heart goes out to all those who have been in the same position.

It was very touch and go over the next 24 hours, but Amy pulled through, I believe, with the help of God. Later I found out that Amy was vomiting up to 15 times a day over the 3 weeks while we were gone. Her system just reacted to the abuse and she collapsed.

Although this was a very traumatic time for me and my family, it did have one very positive outcome. I formulated the method that was about to change everything for us and, more importantly, for Amy. It is not a quick fix, but with dedication, love, and hope, I believe it will work for anyone.

Anorexia and bulimia are not bugs you catch, and they cannot be fixed with a pill. It is a very debilitating psychological problem. Although counseling is an important part of helping beat anorexia in the early stages, when you add the method I've discovered to the treatment, the results will be amazing.

This is my own special way, and it has taken me years of reading, studying, and spending many thousands of dollars to find the answers. Finally, my "Positive Energy Treatment" was born. It worked for Amy, so I do not care about the costs. You can't put a price tag on what it has given me: We got Amy's life back.

Today Amy is a beautiful young woman with the world at her feet. Her weight is a respectable 130 pounds, a far cry from 85 pounds. She has had no symptoms of anorexia or bulimia for at least 2.5 years. Amy now eats 3 regular meals: breakfast, lunch, and dinner. She even eats snacks between main meals, normally fruits or salted biscuits, and sometimes I see her munching on a chocolate as well. We even eat out together once a week and this was something I could only dream about when she was suffering from anorexia and bulimia. Amy has now nearly finished a University course in Psychology and wants to help other people with eating disorders by using the same strategy that I used on her. She is also about to be married to a wonderful young man who has been so supportive of her.

How did Amy and I do it? The next few chapters will explain in detail the steps that Amy and I took for the healing process to begin.

CHAPTER 2

Identifying the Problem: What is an Eating Disorder?

*M*any people just associate this problem with food and/or dieting. But this is not the case. An eating disorder is not about food and dieting.

An eating disorder is a disorder of feelings. For Amy, food abuse helped her respond to her feelings, thus allowing her to avoid, postpone, forget, deny, or otherwise anesthetize her feelings.

For Amy, keeping a safe emotional distance precludes the risk that others will discover her real self and hurt her.

An eating disorder is a disorder of control. Amy perceived that she couldn't control anything in her life except for her food intake and her weight. She perceived that controlling her food in-take and her weight enabled her to keep her uncontrollable life in balance.

An eating disorder is a disorder of thinking. Amy was thinking in a distorted way about herself, the world, and her place in it. She thought that gaining even 1 kilo invariably leads to gaining 10 to 20 kilos.

Her misconception about how she looked is called body image distortion (she thought that she was fat although she was actually very thin). This is also called "broken eye syndrome."

An eating disorder is a disorder of coping. For Amy her eating disorder was the way she coped with everyday stress: with her school, homework, and pressure from her friends.

An eating disorder is a disorder of identity. We realized that Amy had a poor sense of self and the eating disorder became a substitute for her. She described once that being without her disease was unthinkable for her—it was like being without air to breathe. When she was in the hospital, she was afraid that if she recovered, she would "cease to exist."

An eating disorder is a disorder of values and lifestyle. For Amy, spending time with her self and binging was much more important than going out, seeing friends, and socializing.

The eating disorder became her lifestyle, her entertainment, and total interest in life.

An eating disorder is a disorder of relationship. Amy once told one of the counselors: "My best friend is always there for me." This comment was about her eating disorder. She thought of it as her "best friend," her refuge from the hurtful and rejecting people in real life.

When her grandmother died, Amy hid her feelings in her eating disorder. She became very withdrawn and did not want to see anyone or talk to anyone about her pain. She used the eating disorder as an escape; it was better than facing the fact that her grandmother had passed on.

An eating disorder is a disorder of behavior. The extreme unbending and compulsive nature of unbalanced eating behaviors is the main feature of the disease. Amy did not know how to stop. If she eliminated one meal, it would be preferable to eliminate two. If she lost some weight, she would feel that she needed to lose more.

It gave her a form of control she did not normally have in the real world.

CAUSES AND TRIGGERS

The exact cause of eating disorders is not known. However, a combination of factors is believed to contribute to the disease.

Genetic and Biological Factors

Eating disorders seem to run in some families. Women whose mothers or sisters have the disorder are more likely to develop the condition than those who do not have relatives with this problem.

It has also been shown that a single dopamine receptor gene may lie behind the addiction to alcohol, drugs, or food.

Some people carry a form of this pleasure gene, with fewer dopamine receptors. People who inherit this kind of gene may start to use different things like food or alcohol to increase the level of dopamine in the brain.

Psychological Factors

One factor possibly leading to an eating disorder is the way a person looks at the world.

Many theories have been developed to explain how an individual's view of the world may lead to the disorder. It all depends on how a child reacts to bodily changes, life transitions, sexuality issues and how adults react to the stresses of life in general.

Social Influences

Western society places a high value on thinness among women.

Many consider being slim an essential part of beauty and young girls often think that they must be slender to be attractive.

Being thin is also equated with social success. Images of girls and women in the mass media (magazines, television, and movies) have been blamed, in part, for reinforcing such stereotypes.

Some girls become anorexic as a form of copycat behavior. They imitate the actions of other women they admire. Extreme dieting may be one of these behaviors.

Occupational Goals

Some occupations traditionally expect women to be slender. Dancers, fashion models, gymnasts, and actresses are often expected to be very thin. A young girl who aims for these careers may decide to pursue an extreme weight-loss program.

Triggers

Triggers are items or events that spark the beginning of other events.

Eating disorders are often triggered by an event or a circumstance in the life of an individual who is already prone to developing such a condition.

A period of adjustment, such as leaving home to attend summer camp, prep school, or college, can easily trigger disordered eating in an individual with such tendencies already in place.

A traumatic event in someone's life, such as sexual abuse, can also trigger the development of an eating disorder. Other triggers can seem harmless yet represent large life changes, such as moving, starting a new school or job, graduation, and even marriage.

Whatever the trigger is, it is usually closely tied to the end of a valued relationship, or a feeling of loneliness.

The most common trigger of an eating disorder, however, is dieting. Very often, dieting can lead people to disordered eating patterns of some sort, including anorexia or bulimia.

For Amy the trigger probably was initially the death of her grandmother. I suspect it was, although she reacted like she was not upset at all. But I assume it was one type of anorexic behavior, when the individual tries to deny her true feelings by focusing on controlling her food intake.

The final and very substantial trigger was not getting the part in the school dance troupe and believing it was because she was too fat.

Maybe there were other triggers that I don't know because she did not tell me. So if you are a sufferer, look back at your past, and try to see what may have caused your problem. Think all the way back, even to your childhood.

In order to understand how people develop an eating disorder, it's important to recognize that human beings are made up of three components: physical, mental and emotional. (The ancient Greeks talk about people being made up of four components, and include the spiritual. I will assume that the spiritual is something that you can take care of yourself). You can think of it as a triangle:

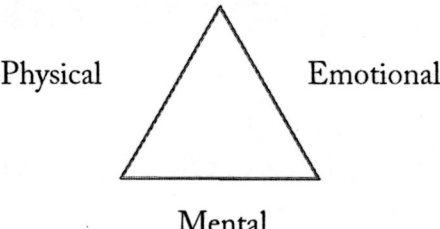

Physical   Emotional

Mental

If any of the three sides is not functioning, the triangle becomes unbalanced.

In healthy people all three sides of the triangle are in balance.

In emotionally vulnerable people (like people with eating disorders), the emotional side becomes unbalanced because of the perceived influence from the outside.

Emotional imbalances start to influence your mental side straight away and then both the emotional and mental start attacking the physical side of the health triangle.

So, what starts as a minor problem in a person who is predisposed to an eating disorder can grow into a major catastrophe, as was the case with Amy not being picked for the dance troupe.

The Method that I applied mainly addresses the emotional component of the triangle. Once the emotional side becomes balanced, it automatically brings the other two sides into balance. (More on this in Chapter 4.)

HOW TO RECOGNIZE SIGNS OF THE DISEASE

How do you recognize the signs of disease? Answering this question can be tricky, as indicators of the disease are generally disguised.

The most accurate assessment will come from your own sensitive and knowledgeable observations of yourself or loved one.

If you are on your own, you will have to be brutally honest with yourself and answer the questions truthfully—even if it will hurt you emotionally to do so. If you are reading this book, you're past step one and have acknowledged the problem, so be honest for the rest of the treatment.

Here is the list of signs for the disease. In hindsight, I noticed that Amy had these in the early stages of her eating disorder.

1. Excessive and rapid weight loss
2. Poor self-image
3. Do you feel fat even though you are actually thin? Can you describe fat as a feeling?

4. Do you deny hunger?

5. Do you only eat a limited variety of foods: like raw vegetables, low fat yogurts, cereal, raw fruits and bananas?

6. Has your period stopped and has it been absent for months or years?

7. Do you exercise a lot, up to 3-5 hours a day?

8. Do you weigh yourself daily, sometimes a few times a day?

9. Do you use laxatives excessively?

10. Amy's counselor told me that Amy was dreaming about food, even when she was going to bed and was trying to fall asleep. She was dreaming about different foods she could eat. Do you do the same thing?

11. Do you refuse to eat in front of others? For this reason, do you avoid parties, friend's dinners, and the like?

12. Do you run off and disappear to the bathroom a lot, especially after meals?

13. Do you have extreme mood swings? Most of the time this is a big sign that you have an eating disorder.

14. Do you believe your life would be much better if you were thinner, even though people tell you you are already thin?

15. Do you avoid personal intimate connections with people?

16. Are you obsessed with the size of your clothes and believe the smaller the size of clothes you have, the better?

17. Most of the time Amy felt very vulnerable. She distrusted herself and others. If you feel like this then you are definitely in the danger zone.

HOW TO TALK TO YOUR CHILD (OR LOVED ONE)

The closer people are to you, the more influence you get from them. So it is important for any caretaker or person close to the sufferer not to make judgments.

An eating disorder suggests that a person's developmental thinking (concerning relationships, coping strategies, self-communication, and self-evaluation) have gone off track.

If you have suspicions that your loved one has an eating disorder, go face to face with your loved one and talk to them. Again if you are on your own, be honest with yourself.

I was watching once on a daytime television talk show about how to deal with kids with eating disorder. Many parents from the audience were able to say the right words, even without a clear understanding of how the mind actually works. But at least they knew how to act.

The suggestions they gave were not to "nag" children. Don't force them to eat or attempt to control their food. This is the same for adults.

Some of them mention that what you have to offer to your loved one is her/his "self-esteem," not food. Just love the child and offer unconditional love. This is exactly the same for adults.

When you are approaching an adult to talk about their eating disorder you should be prepared to enter a volatile and uncertain situation. Especially if they have not admitted they have a problem.

Your loved one may put you off by their responses. They may say things like: "I don't feel like talking now," or "I keep it all under control," or just denies the problem all together.

She may also be very embarrassed by the question you ask and reject you.

When the conversation comes to a dead end, take the initiative to finish it in a natural way. Don't get angry and don't leave with statements like, "I give up," "I don't care anymore," or "You are on your own."

Tell them that you love them very much and you will continue to do so, and that it doesn't matter what they do. Tell them that you are open to helping them at any time they decide to come to you. Tell them that you wish you can help and will do everything possible to help them get better.

Make yourself unconditionally available for help. So, when they feel like they can come and talk to you heart to heart, you are there for them.

Never judge, never snap, or do anything similar to these.

Only this approach (from love and a caring point of view) will make your loved one comfortable enough to talk to you about his/her problems.

Parents are teachers. Parents teach children about life and how to live it.

If the conversation becomes problematic, in a calm, loving voice, tell your child: "I love you. It doesn't matter what you do and because I love you, I also must take care of you. I want to be your friend—not your enemy—and I am always on your side. And because I am on your side I want you to be well and not suffer any longer. I want you to know that I will always be on your side—not on anyone else's."

MY DIALOGUE WITH AMY

I remember when I started my first serious conversation with Amy about her eating habits. When I found out we had a big problem, the conversation went like this:

Me: I am concerned about you. Here is what I have observed: you have not been eating and you are so thin. I have noticed you have just been chewing your food but not swallowing it. Also, I found a lot of empty boxes of laxatives when I was cleaning your room. I'm just very concerned that there is something wrong with you. You know, I am your mother and I love you dearly and I don't want anything happening to you. What do you think about all these things?

Amy: It's really none of your business.

Me: I understand what you think, but I really want to know more about how you arrived at this conclusion. The problem I have noticed might possibly be a matter of your health. I think maybe a professional should help us to determine what it is and what we can do to help."

Amy: I am not going to see anyone because there is nothing wrong with me; I keep everything under control.

Me: I see that this situation scares you and makes you feel out of control. A lot of people who don't understand eating disorders think all sorts of scary things about them, like once you have a disorder you have got it for life. But you know that these notions are not true.

Amy: Of course. I also know there is nothing wrong with me. I am just trying to keep my weight under control so I can look good.

Me: Eating disorders are a very confusing problem. It seems to be about food and weight, but generally they are about your feelings, your thoughts, coping mechanisms, anxiety, and relationships. And if you are out of control with your food, you are probably feeling out of control with other things as well. Eating disorders reflect how a person thinks, acts, and feels in general.

Amy: Okay, so let's say I have a problem and I went for help. What can they do for me and what happens if nothing helps me to get better? Then what?

Me: I understand your concern, because eating disorder recovery can take some time and can be quite challenging. But I want you to know that I am going to support you in any situation as long as it's needed. You will need to go through a few changes in the way you feel, think, and react.

Amy: I am not ready to get help now; I don't think there is a problem. I'll take care of this next week. I just need to finish my science project in time. Maybe next week I will go for it.

Me: You know, the longer you wait, the more damage you can do to your body. It is much better to treat the disease in the early stages.

Amy: I promise that I can make a few changes myself. I really don't need anybody's help.

Me: My dear Amy, if you had asthma and needed regular puffers to control your asthma, I would be responsible as your parent to make sure you got the medical attention you needed. Now I think you have an eating disorder, so I want to make sure that you get all the medical help that is necessary for it. What if I offer you a hand, just temporarily, until you are free to take control of things on your own again? What do you think about that?

Amy: I guess that sounds fair. I just wish I could be good enough the way I am.

Me: You are certainly good enough. I really want you to stay that way.

If you are dealing with an adult, then you may have to adjust the questions a little, but it is still a relevant format. Remember, an adult may use stronger language than a child would use, but do not get angry. It will not do any good, and will probably make things worse, and the sufferer will not want to confide in you.

If you have no one to help you, then ask yourself the same questions. You already know you have a problem; just be honest with yourself.

HOW TO EMPOWER YOURSELF TO COPE WITH YOUR—OR YOUR LOVED ONE'S—CONDITION

If you or the person you are trying to help still cannot acknowledge the problem, then:

- Understand that you (and the person close to you) are not responsible for your illness (like any illness), BUT it is your responsibility and your decision to improve and even cure yourself. Without this decision, nothing and nobody can help.

- Try to contact other people who have the same problem and talk to them about treatment methods, but not about how to conceal your problem.

- Talk to counselors or psychologists about your worries and anxieties. They can help in the early stages to get you to admit you have a problem. Don't let them talk you into years of group therapy or counseling, as this does not work. Think of it this way: if it did work, then why does it take years? Remember it is their job and they get paid to do it. If they had no one to counsel, then they would not get paid. But they can help in the early stages to root out the cause of the problem.

- Read as much as possible about eating disorders. The more you know about the disease, the easier it becomes to conquer it.

CHAPTER 3

The Method: What is Positive Energy Treatment?

"The secret of the method was what enabled us to help Amy recover from her eating disorder. I believe that not understanding this secret was the reason we could not succeed when we were initially trying to help her —and it cost her many years of suffering."

No doctor told me about the method I discovered, and the information wasn't in any of the mainstream literature. The method is "Positive Energy Treatment."

You have to change your subconscious mind to change your feelings, thoughts, and identity.

I already mentioned earlier that eating disorders are disorders of feelings, thoughts, identity, values, relationships, coping and control.

And if you fix all of the above or change these feelings to new ones (like positive feelings and thoughts, a strong sense of identity and values, good coping and control strategies, high self-esteem), only then will you be able to recover from an eating disorder quickly.

I have been told by some people who are sufferers, when I talk to them, that they already know all this. My question to them is simple: If you do, then why are you still a sufferer? It is obvious that they have missed something important and should try again, this time with an open mind.

I discovered a few special ways to reach your own subconscious mind:

1. Playing the game "Who are you?" to realize true identity
2. Using power words for positive affirmations
3. Using progressive relaxation techniques
4. Using a gratitude exercise every morning to get new values in your life or replace old values
5. Laughing an hour every day to change your feelings to something more positive
6. Building a dream board to help you change your focus—from controlling your eating to controlling your future
7. Learning to believe in yourself
8. Creating new mental associations and perceptions
9. Eliminating limiting beliefs

10. Using modern technology for anorexia-bulimia treatment
11. Giving gratitude

If you are helping a child under 18, the special ways to reach their subconscious mind would be a little bit different. Here is what I did with Amy (she was under 18 when I had first discovered the disease):

1. Playing the game "Who are you?"
2. Using power words for positive affirmations
3. Using progressive relaxation technique.
4. Talking about values a lot at home. If the children wanted, they can contribute to the discussion, but we did not force them to participate. It helped to change Amy's way of thinking even though she did not initially want to be involved.
5. Laughing an hour every day for many years
6. Building a dream board
7. Learning to believe in yourself
8. Creating new mental associations and perceptions
9. Eliminating limiting beliefs
10. Finding and changing emotional triggers around the home

I should say that influencing anyone's subconscious mind is not a quick process. It takes time. But if you are persistent, you will definitely see a significant improvement in your mental state within a few weeks to a few months after beginning the exercises above. It all depends on the individual.

Again, I have been told by some sufferers that they know all this and have even tried it before. But if you feel like this, then you have not grasped the significance of the aforementioned 11 exercises. If you did, you would not be reading this book.

How does it work, you ask?

Here is the short and simple explanation. Our brain consists of two halves (called hemispheres). Both hemispheres are covered by a thick layer called the cortex. The cortex is the conscious part of the brain, the part we think with (just logic thinking). But this part of the brain is not responsible for our feelings.

We have another small part of our brain, which lies between the two hemispheres and connects them. This little part is called the limbic system. The limbic system, as discussed in the next section, is involved in regulating emotions and motivations. In addition, parts of the limbic system, the amygdala and hippocampus, are important for memory.

The limbic system does not have consciousness (or thoughts, only feelings). In other words, the limbic system is what we call our subconscious, or subconscious mind.

It has been found that people with emotional problems have an imbalance of the limbic system or subconscious. This includes problems like anxiety, depression, eating disorders, alcoholism, and other addictions.

In the period of acute stress, we also have an imbalance in the limbic system (or subconscious)—that is why stress affects us, not only emotionally, but mentally and physically.

After stress, some people recover quickly—and we call them "strong people." What "strong" actually means is that they know how to affect their limbic system (subconscious) and put it in balance.

The question is: How do you influence the limbic system and put it in the right balance?

The answer: The cortex, which is the conscious part of the brain, should influence the limbic system, which does not have conscious thought. The cortex, which makes decisions, learns new things, and understands things for us, should influence the non-conscious part of the brain by giving signals to the limbic system to work differently.

Most eating disorders are a learned behavior. Initially you taught yourself to diet, or to become slim. Initially it was your own conscious decision to lose weight because you wanted to look better. This conscious decision was made by your cortex and sent to your limbic system, which gave you feelings (like feeling good about yourself when you become slim).

So, what you need to do is reverse this; you (or your cortex) should make another decision (about changing your own image and feelings that you have now, like starving yourself or purging, back to a normal response) and send this signal to your limbic system to foster good feelings about this new decision you have just made.

How do you do it? There are lots of examples on how this works. There are special new programs that can automatically affect the limbic system of your brain (the part of the brain where the eating disorder lives). These programs can identify and eliminate your subconscious blockages that created your eating disorder in the first place. You will get the information about one of these special new programs later in the book.

But now, I will describe to you the strategies I used to treat my daughter Amy. And because of them, she recovered and now lives a beautiful and fulfilling life.

PART 1: THE SECRET GAME—"WHO ARE YOU?"

This game really helped Amy to find her identity. She obviously had very poor self-esteem, and the eating disorder became a substitute for her "self." She often described to me the internal emptiness, like having a hole in her chest.

If you have suffered from anorexia or bulimia for a while, you're probably familiar with the feelings of emptiness inside when you think that there is nothing really much in your life—except for the great feeling of weird satisfaction that you get from binging or starving yourself. You may even sometimes think: "What if there is no eating disorder? What would I do with my life? How would I satisfy myself? How would I feel in control still? How would I live?"

But don't worry. These are common thoughts of eating disorder sufferers, and you can easily get rid of them if you know how.

Remember, eating disorder sufferers (at least a majority of them) are gifted and talented people. They get an eating disorder because they are perfectionists. They don't want to be anything except perfect. They want to have perfect bodies as well—and that is why they get an eating disorder. Eating disorders are really an exaggerated response to trying to lose some weight.

Now, how to do the exercise

This exercise should become one of your rituals. Practice the following exercise at least three times a week, in the morning or before going to bed, for at least the first three weeks.

Preparing for the exercise:

- You can turn on a meditation tape on low volume for background music if you want to during the exercise, but it is not necessary, although it can help your mind relax and be more receptive (to reach an Alpha state).

- It is preferable to do simple relaxation for at least 10 minutes before you start doing the exercise, because you can't get access to your subconscious mind if you are not in a relaxed state. You can just listen to soft music for 10 minutes before this exercise.

- If you find it hard to relax, just think about something pleasant. Think of a nice moment before the eating disorder happened and dwell on this for a while (In the next chapter, there are a few suggestions on how to relax by just listening).

Beginning the exercise:

- If you have no one to help you, you should sit in front of a mirror. Look directly into your eyes. Relax as much as you can and ask the questions in a very quiet, monotonous voice to the person you see in the mirror. Of course, if you have a partner or a loved one to help you, it is easier to do it with that person.

Now, if you are doing this by yourself, you have to imagine that the person looking back at you is a different person and not you. This person is your sounding board for this exercise.

The first question you should ask yourself is: "Who are you?" You should ask this question every 20-30 seconds. Ask this question until an answer comes to mind. Write the answer down (especially the answer that first comes to your mind). The first answer is normally the correct one as it comes from your subconscious mind. If you think about the answer, or change it to your second thought, then this comes from your thinking mind and it will probably be untrue.

The question "Who are you?" should be repeated every 20-30 seconds for 3 minutes. All answers should be recorded (on a piece of paper or sound recorder, if you want). A sound recorder is better because you do not lose your concentration.

At first, this exercise seems a bit strange to do, but when you get the hang of it, it works really well. You should not make any comments or prompt yourself when you do it. You should listen to your subconscious mind.

The person who is helping you should not make comments either; they should simply ask the question. If someone is helping, get them to remember what you said and talk about it later.

After asking "Who are you?" do the same with the question "What do you want?"

Ask this question every 20-30 seconds, looking into your eyes in the mirror while you do so, for at least three minutes. Write down all your own answers, and evaluate your answers after at least five days of doing this exercise.

And the last question is: "What is your purpose?" Follow the same procedure.

Again, if you have a person to help you out, it is much more comfortable to do. If you do have someone to help you, they can interact with you by directly asking you the questions, but they must not make judgment, or prompt you in anyway. They should just ask the questions ("Who are you?", "What do you want?" and "What is your purpose?") in a monotone voice.

If there is a helper, you can rotate the questions. First the helper, then the sufferer, but the helper should not overreact with the answers; they must be genuine.

Summary:

Ask yourself three questions:

"Who are you?"   every 20-30 sec for three minutes

"What do you want?"   every 20-30 sec for three minutes

"What is your purpose?" every 20-30 sec for three minutes

After doing this exercise for at least five times, sit down and think about your answers. Don't judge yourself too hard. There are no right or wrong answers. The results only show you the perceptions you have of yourself up to that point.

You can change your answers; replace them with new ones if you want at anytime. You will find that, over time, the answers will change naturally as you progress.

Some of you will notice that you can put yourself in a hypnotic trance quite easily, although it may not happen right away, or at the first attempt. (It is really a hypnotic experience to stare at your reflection—looking straight into your eyes—and asking the same questions repeatedly.)

If you are on your own please use hypnotic music or a hypnotic CD before you do this, as it takes more concentration to do this when doing it by yourself. The more relaxed you are, the better. Some of you may take longer to fully access your own subconscious mind, but it will come with more and more practice.

When I say hypnosis you should not think it is something like a hypnotic show you see on TV. The only thing I did is described above—no gimmicky stuff like on TV. That is entertainment; this is totally different. It is the feeling you get during this exercise that is very special and can be only compared to a hypnotic experience.

Later on, when answering the questions becomes easy, add on more complicated questions like:

"Do you want to change?"

"How are you going to change?"

"What do you want to do to change?"

I did this exercise with Amy for a long time, actually, for more than a year, every day. What did it do? This exercise helped Amy to identify herself—who she really was, what she wanted and what her real purpose in life was.

Of course, I had to help her do it, but she was only a child who needed to be helped.

The main purpose of this exercise is to identify where you are now and where you want to go.

Don't worry about your answers. If they are not what you would like to hear, you can change that with the help of the other exercises that I will explain to you later.

During this exercise you will probably find out something about yourself that you never thought about before.

You may find out that you do not feel safe and perceive the world to be a very hostile place—this alone could be a reason for your mental escape in the form of your eating disorder.

So, the goal is to change your own thoughts, feelings and perceptions on a subconscious level, but it takes time, especially for someone who has eating problems.

PART 2: CHANGING YOUR VOCABULARY

Think about the vocabulary you normally use in your every day language. What words do you pronounce again and again every day? Are these positive and well-meaning words? Or do you use a lot of negative words that mean failure, doubt, insecurity, or have other negative meanings?

Why do I ask this? All words (used in conversation with others or just with yourself) have energy and power.

If you use a lot of negative words like "I can't do it," "It is bad," "It never works," "I don't like it," "I feel bad," "I am tired," "I have no energy," "I am not good enough," "I am sick," "I will never change," "Nothing makes me happy," or something similar, you send a signal to the Universe about what you want and the Universe just gives you back all the negatives. You have heard the old saying "like attracts like." If you live in a world of negative, then there is zero chance that anything positive will come along.

So, what do you think you will end up with? You will end up with the same old bad feelings, of course. The very same old feelings that you have been trying to mask by starving yourself, or binging and purging.

You see, unless you change these old feelings and start to send the Universe new signals—with better meanings—by using more positive language, like "I can," "It always works," and "Things happen for the better," it will be harder to change your negative association with food.

Conclusion:

Stop using all negative words in your vocabulary altogether, and replace them with positive, powerful, and well-meaning ones.

The powerful words I suggest that you start using every day are: peace, harmony, freedom, love, inspiration, guidance, health, vitality, power, strength, confidence, wisdom, energy, abundance, honesty, kindness, "I can do anything," "I like it," "I believe it," "I feel great," "I am so grateful," "It's my pleasure," "I'm excited," "It's amazing," "It's wonderful," and more.

Please, continue my list of positive words that you can use in your everyday language.

Note: Use the words above every day, as many times as you can for at least a 6-month period.

PART 3: CHANGING YOUR SELF-TALK USING CONSTRUCTIVE AFFIRMATIONS

Perform this exercise in a relaxed emotional state because the affirmation you are going to use should reach your subconscious mind.

You will have to explain this part to the child more carefully.

It is recommended to do at least three minutes of relaxation before you start to do constructive affirmation. (See three-minute relaxation technique in the next chapter).

The best way to do affirmation, in my opinion, is doing constructive affirmations. What this means:

- Take a piece of paper and draw a vertical line down the middle of it.
- On the left side you should start writing personal affirmation, or goals from the 1st person (start with I):

Examples:

"I am feeling happy eating three average size meals a day"

"I have an abundance of strength to get good health."

"I love my body as it is, nice and proportionate."

When you write your sentence on the left side of the paper, try to feel what your subconscious mind says to you at this moment. (This is the little voice inside your head that always says you can't do something.) Your subconscious mind may say "No way" at first. Write this answer on the right side of the paper, opposite the sentence on the left side.

Write this affirmation as many times as you can on the left side of the paper and always write the answer from your subconscious mind on the right side. But try to persuade your subconscious mind to accept your "I am feeling happy eating three average size meals a day."

By the end of the page, your subconscious mind may start giving you more positive answers.

After doing affirmations from the first person perspective "I", write the same affirmation but from a second person perspective: "You."

Examples:

"You are feeling happy eating three average size meals a day."

"You have an abundance of strength to get good health."

"You love your body as it is, nice and proportionate."

And also listen to your subconscious mind and write your answers on the right side, opposite the sentences on the left.

But always try to persuade your subconscious mind to accept the meaning of the sentence: "You are feeling happy eating three averagesize meals a day."

In the beginning of this exercise your subconscious mind may say, "No you can't feel happy," but in the end, the answer you get should change to something more positive.

Then write the same affirmations from a third person perspective: "She" or "He."

"She is feeling happy eating three average size meals a day."

"She has an abundance of strength to get good health."

"She loves her body as it is, nice and proportionate."

And the same procedure applies; write the answers from your subconscious mind on the right side of the paper, opposite the sentences on the left.

When you write these affirmations from a third person perspective, "She," you should imagine that you are talking about yourself like you are a different "third" person, and look at yourself from that third person point of view.

You can do any personal affirmation or goals this way. You can adjust them according to your situation and circumstances.

What this exercise does is change the perception of your subconscious mind in relation to food and feelings. Also, constructive affirmations put you in an emotional state where eating and emotional problems are not an issue.

All the time you do the affirmation, you order your subconscious mind to act like you do not have any eating or emotional problems.

The more often you do it, the quicker the results and faster the healing.

I would recommend you do it each day for the next 30 days. If you manage to do it for this period of time, I am sure you'll see a positive change in your life. You will be amazed at how you will feel. Your feelings and relationship with food will improve.

When to use constructive affirmations:

Do constructive affirmations when you have free 10-15 minutes during your lunch break, or any time in the middle of day.

Here are more examples of positive affirmations you can use for changing your self-talk (but use them in the 1st, 2nd, and 3rd person: I, you and she/he).

"I want to find inner peace; I will find inner peace."

"I am happy to have dinner with my family."

"I have freedom of choice and a lot of power to stop my eating disorder."

"I am inspired, looking to my bright future."

"I have an abundance of strength to get good health."

"I live in harmony with my own self."

"I have an abundance of energy."

You can make up your own affirmations using positive power words described in Part 2.

PART 4: USING PROGRESSIVE RELAXATION TECHNIQUES

One of the ways to reach your subconscious mind is relaxation, which helps you to relieve tension and free your mind from obsessive thoughts.

Before doing the exercise "Who are you?" and doing constructive affirmations, it is good to relax. If you are not in the relaxed emotional state, you will not be able to communicate with your subconscious mind and get the right answers.

As an eating disorder sufferer, you've probably noticed that it is not easy for you to relax because most of the time you worry about something, feel restless, or obsess with needless thoughts. Am I right?

Amy was very tense initially, and did not respond to relaxation at first. But I continued to teach her this relaxation technique over and over again. I did not know much about relaxation before; I just started to read on how to do it, learned it myself, and then taught Amy.

Here is a very simple meditation-relaxation technique I used to help Amy:

Find an area in your home where you can have about three minutes to yourself. That's right, you only need three minutes in your quest for success. After practicing this exercise many times, you may reduce the time to only one or two minutes.

Now read the following words into a recording device.

Read very, very slowly. Pretend that you are tired as you read this exercise and you will react in a relaxed, sleepy manner.

Start reading:

"Sit up in a comfortable chair or lie on a couch or bed with your hands resting on your lap or by your side ….take two slow deep breaths….each time you inhale, focus on filling your lungs with clean, fresh air…..as you exhale, feel all the tension leave your lungs. You feel good, you feel fine…..you feel perfectly relaxed.

Each and every deep breath that you take lets you relax deeper and deeper ….each and every sound that you hear allows you to relax deeper and deeper ….nothing will disturb you….just breathe deeply and relax deeply….Let your body relax….let all of your muscles relax as you gain control over the powerful subconscious part of your mind ….all of your cares and troubles are just drifting away…. You can bring them back any time you want …but it feels good to let them drift away at this time…

Each and every breath you take allows you to relax deeper and deeper…Each and every sound you hear allows you relax deeper and deeper…You feel good, you feel fine …you feel perfect and complete…Your brain is alert and aware and your body is relaxing perfectly…Each and every time I practice this exercise, I will find myself relaxing to a greater and greater degree…

My body feels totally relaxed as my mind is keenly alert, aware and very powerful…I can achieve anything I want when I execute my own mind power…I will find myself sleeping better when it's time to sleep and I will find more energy when I am awake…My life is getting better and better…

Day by day, in every way, I am getting better and better. I feel good…I feel fine…I feel totally and completely relaxed… In a moment I am going to count from 1 to 5 …By the time I reach 5, I will be alert and awake and feeling better than I have ever felt before…Each and every time I practice this exercise, I will find myself relaxing to a greater and greater degree…all right …one…two…three…four…FIVE…I am wide awake…alert and feeling better in every way."

This relaxation technique you can use any time you need it, especially when you get uptight or stressed.

Don't worry if your thoughts still wander when you are trying to relax. Just continue to do it over and over again. Eventually you will relax automatically when you start listening to your recorded voice.

You can also use this little mantra while you relax if all the thoughts keep running around in your head. It is OOMM NA MA SHAVIA. Just keep repeating this over and over again, and you will be able to control your wayward thoughts and relax.

PART 5: BUILDING A DREAM BOARD

Building a dream board is one of the more important parts of the secret I discovered. My whole family participated in building a dream board.

And don't think that building a dream board is just for children. Don't think it is silly because it is not and is really important.

For adults it is necessary to have your own dream board; you put everything you want the Universe to give you on this board.

What is a dream board, you may ask? Well, here is what you do, and it is very simple.

You need a big peace of cardboard (I had 50cm by 70cm) for each participant.

You need old magazines and/or brochures with lots of pictures of all sorts of different things in it. You need glue and scissors.

Everyone then looks through the magazines and cuts out photos and things they would love to have, or places they would love to go, or what they would really like to do.

The dream board is made by gluing as many photos of things you want on the cardboard, in no particular order (but it has to be things you are dreaming about).

The cardboard can be any color you like. Except black or gray.

Again, on your dream board, you should show what you dream about.

For example, what house you want to live in, what car you want to drive, what kind of furniture you want to have, what places you want to visit, what dresses you want to wear, how you see yourself in the future, what you want to do in the future, how you are going to feel in the future.

You should continue doing it until all your dream board is full of pictures and all the pictures represent your dreams and hopes for the future.

After you finish the board, you put it up on the wall in your bedroom or somewhere where you can see it all the time to remind yourself about your dreams and what you really desire.

It was a fantastic opportunity for Amy to start dreaming about the future and focus on that future instead of her eating disorder.

Why this works so well is while you are doing it, you are in a relaxed state and thinking about all the positive things you want out of life. You are in an alpha brain wave pattern, so all your desires go straight to your subconscious mind. This is where the real battle with eating disorders must be fought and won. (More on alpha brain waves later in the book).

Although we all were doing it together, it is really a very personal experience because your dream board is what you want in life.

No one is telling you what you should put on your board. These are your dreams and your future hopes that you want that go on the board.

After building the dream boards, I actually realized that Amy had a lot of ambitions and wanted a lot of things for herself.

I think it was the first time, in a real way, we got Amy to look at a positive future.

I also made it a ritual for everyone to look at their dream boards every day, and to reflect on what their dreams are.

I truly believe that building the dream board was a major step in Amy's rehabilitation and, for a short while, while building it, she was free from her demons.

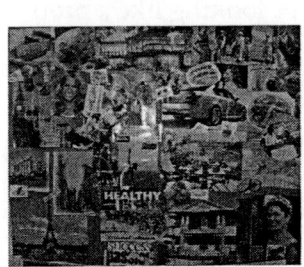

Amy's dream board

You don't have to have other people with you to make your own dream board. As I said, it is a personal experience and doing it on your own is as good as doing with someone else.

I think when you do it by yourself, you even have more time and fewer distractions so you may concentrate and think about what you want in life.

Looking at your dream board daily will make you focus on the things you want to have and achieve in your live. This will take your focus from food and weight loss to what is really important in your life.

I know from correspondences we get that many people do not do the dream board for some reason. Whether they think it is childish, I am not sure, but it is very important, so please do it. I don't recommend things if they are not important. The program is meant to be followed, as it is important in attacking the mental blockages in your subconscious mind—but more on that later.

PART 6: LAUGHING AN HOUR EVERY DAY

Yes, we did it. I tried to find as many jokes as possible to make everyone laugh at home. Laughter is one of the things that affects your subconscious mind very positively.

We all tried to make and find jokes, including jokes about an eating disorder. I think jokes, especially about eating disorders, helped Amy to feel more relaxed about her condition, accept it, and then slowly let it go.

If you can laugh about something, it stops looking like a problem. If the problem is not a problem anymore, you will let go of it with ease.

At first, Amy was a bit offended by eating disorders and dieting jokes, but later she just laughed.

I think that these jokes helped her to accept the problem and face it.

I noticed a big difference in how Amy felt after each time we had a good laugh. She was just more alive and smiling, and it looked like she returned to her normal self before the eating disorder state.

I would suggest that you watch as much comedy on TV or at the movies as you can. If it is funny, just laugh and don't worry about anyone else or what they may think. You are doing it for you, no one else.

Here are some special jokes from my list (eating disorder jokes). They are not meant to offend; so just laugh at them.

1. Wife to her overweight husband: Last night there were two pieces of cake in this pantry and now there is only one. How do you explain that?
   Husband: I guess it was so dark that I didn't see the other piece.

2. The biggest drawback to fasting for seven days is that it makes one "weak."

3. Most people gain weight by having intimate dinners for two...alone.

4. A diet is what you go on when not only can you fit into store dresses; you can't fit in the dressing room as well

5. One guideline applies to fat and thin people alike: If you're thin, don't eat fast. If you're fat, don't eat—FAST.

6. Whether you want to be thick or thin IS A MATTER OF TASTE!!!

7. SKINNY PEOPLE TICK ME OFF!!! Especially when they say things like, "You know, sometimes I forget to eat." Now I've forgotten my address, my mother's maiden name, and my car keys, but I have never forgotten to eat. You have to be a special kind of stupid to forget to eat.

8. He took the doctor's advice too far.

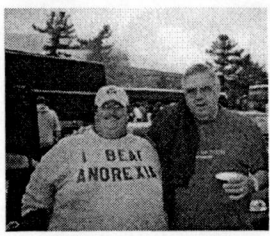

I suggest you look for jokes like these in papers, magazines or books. You definitely can use any jokes you like (not only about eating disorders). The important thing is you have to have a good laugh at least once in a week, but more often is better.

Eating disorder jokes will help you see a funny side to your condition, so your brain starts changing the way it perceives your eating disorder.

"Laughter attracts joy, releases negativity, and leads to miraculous cures."

-Rhonda Byrne

PART 7: LEARNING TO BELIEVE IN YOURSELF

Most eating disorder sufferers have low self-esteem. They also have a false perception that only skinny people are good and successful. They get totally preoccupied with these kinds of thoughts.

Moreover, they believe that without their eating disorder, they can't achieve other things in life that they wish to achieve.

This happened to Amy, too. She thought that controlling her food intake was her way to survive in this world. After building the dream board, we realized that Amy had many ambitions and dreams. And it was very good and reassuring at that stage.

The next problem was how to make the dreams come true if she had an eating disorder.

You know that an eating disorder takes all your energy, focus, and time. Eating disorders make you aloof and withdrawn from people. You stop socializing and meeting new people because of the fear of being forced to eat something.

You much prefer to spend time alone to binge and purge, make a new restrictive diet plan, or calculate your calorie intake and exercise to the extreme if you decide that "you have been eating too much."

Does it sound familiar? Does it sound like someone you know?

At this point, you really have to decide on what you want to do: continue to starve yourself or binge and purge, or start building a new life full of meaning, purpose, and contribution.

Make your choice now! You are putting your life up on a stage, and pointing to where your life will go. This is the crossroads. Is it back to misery and failure, or towards happiness and success? It is your choice; right here, right now, choose.

A great quote by Henry Ford says, "If you think you can or you think you can't, you are always right."

I constantly repeated these words to Amy when we had conversations about losers and winners and their different approaches to life.

Read what a famous singer, Paula Abdul, said in this regard:

"Overcoming an eating disorder myself has made me prouder than selling millions of albums."

Winning a battle with an eating disorder is a big success in anyone's life. But in reality, this winning requires only two things: believing that you are a winner and feeling that you are already a winner.

Now imagine that you don't have an eating disorder—that you eat the normal three meals a day, don't purge, and don't work off the calories to excess. Imagine that you lost the focus on food and weight loss. What would your life be like?

Can you see your new image?

Hold this new image of the new you in your head and feel it.

Now, stand up for a minute and walk around the room with feelings of the new you (think you have beaten your eating disorder completely).

Without any doubt, this feels fantastic! Did you notice how you walk now: with confidence and open shoulders, your back is straight, and your eyes look enlightened?

Don't lose these feelings; keep them for as long as you can until these feelings become a habit.

To keep and maintain a winner's attitude, you should take a whole winner's approach to life. This is the secret to winning against your eating disorder.

Here's a list of how losers and winners approach their life and how they react in different situations:

Losers approach life with an "Oh, poor me" attitude (the victim mentality).
Winners approach life with an enthusiastic "I can do it!!!" attitude.

Losers expect to fail before they even start.
Winners live life with the positive expectation about their own success and the success of others.

Losers give up when things get tough.
Winners turn every situation (even tough ones) into a positive and expect to solve the problem as they arrive.

Losers always think negatively about themselves and others.
Winners always think positively about themselves and others.
Losers face each day aimlessly with no real purpose in life.
Winners know where they are going, and there is purpose in everything they do. (In time Amy finally understood that everything we were doing had a purpose—to stop her eating disorder and achieve the dreams she wanted).

Losers always expect something for nothing.
Winners are willing to pay the price and make the sacrifice to get results. (Amy in the end finally understood that she had to beat her eating disorder to achieve the dreams she wished).

Losers worry about what cannot be done.
Winners focus on what can be done and how to make it happen.
(Amy soon understood that what we were doing could be done and it started to take her focus away from her eating disorder).

Losers blame others and make excuses when they fail.
Winners accept responsibility and learn lessons from each experience.

Losers put themselves and others down.
Winners expect the best from others and from themselves.

Losers give up on their dreams.
Winners think big, dream big, and follow their dreams.

Losers never give 100% to what they do.
Winners always give 110% to what they do.
Losers are quitters and never win.
Winners never quit and persist until they succeed.

Can you see how changing the focus away from the eating disorder starts to have a profound effect on you?

You have to believe that you are a winner who has already won the battle against your eating disorder because:

"For those who believe,
no proof is necessary.
For those who don't believe,
no proof is possible."

- John & Lyn St. Clair Thomas, "Eyes of the Beholder"

You only need to change your state of mind to beat your eating disorder and stay on the high emotional stage to continue to be free of it.

Always look after your emotional state—this is a key to your success.

"Until you can understand that nothing can
happen to you, nothing can ever come to you, or
be kept from you, except in accord with your state
of consciousness, you do not have the key to life."

- Paul Twitchell

PART 8: CREATING NEW MENTAL ASSOCIATIONS AND PERCEPTIONS

An eating disorder sufferer associates all their good, positive feelings of control, pleasure, truth, and self-confidence with food. She feels reassured by the control she has over her food intake and uses it as a substitute for her lack of control over their true feelings in the real world.

So, the question is: How do you go about changing these distorted associations with food? What must be done exactly to get the sufferer to see other avenues for herself? How do you change her present condition and misdirected dependence on food? More importantly, can we get the sufferer to change at all?

The answer is: yes, we can.

But how can we do it? We need to change the meaning she has attached to food, to break the endless cycle she finds herself in and create a totally different one. Difficult, yes, but not impossible.

Actually, all successes attributed to psychotherapy only ever depend on how quickly people can change the meaning they attach to different things in life.

Here are three fundamentals to create a new meaning in life (in the case of eating disorder sufferers, this is about food and control):

1. **Get leverage.** This means you have to get to the point where you believe you must change your eating habits and you MUST change them right now. You must believe that not changing will be more painful and that changing will bring you pleasure.

If you only get to the point of thinking that you maybe should change, well, this is not enough to create a long-lasting change in your behavior. Only a definite MUST change will give you leverage over the eating disorder.

2. **Interrupt the pattern.** This is when you do something totally unexpected in relation to your dominant thoughts, in our case, food.

For example, when a bulimic person gets a bit stressed by the end of the day, or feels uncomfortable regarding something, the first thought and reaction for her would be binge eating and purging. This is her way of getting pleasure, control, and inner confidence.

For anorexics, the thoughts of success, looking good, and being confident are associated with refusing to eat and starving themselves. This is their way of dealing with things.

This pattern (of thought association) needs to be interrupted with some unexpected comment or behavior that shocks the person into paying more attention to what is going on right here and now in her mind.

For example, I watched on cable TV once how one American psychotherapist goes about breaking the thought patterns of people with major phobias. One man had a major phobia with spiderswas horrified just thinking about them.

The Psychotherapist asked the guy, "How do you feel about spiders?"

The man turned pale and looked extremely anxious, and his answer was, "Not very good...." And at this particular moment, the psychotherapist jumped from his chair and started hopping on one foot in front of the man, shouting very loudly "Yam, yam, yam, yam," and making jerky and funny movements with his whole body.

The man looked stunned, his attention was 100% on the psychotherapist now; he forgot instantly about his scared feelings toward spiders.

After jumping and shouting for a minute, the psychotherapist stopped, sat on his chair like nothing had happened.

After a small pause he asks the man again how he felt about spiders. The man did not answer straight away because he actually needed a few seconds more to bring himself to the state of spider phobia again.

During the few seconds when the man was thinking, the psychotherapist repeated what he did the first time, making the man completely confused about what was going on.

The Psychotherapist repeated the whole procedure quite a few times (5 or 6).

What do you think happened to the man? He was completely cured of his phobia, just from one single psychotherapy section.

3. **Breaking the old associations.** An interview with this man taken a few months later was shown on TV as well. In this interview, he said he does not have fear spiders anymore.

He also said that now, if someone mentions spiders to him, he laughs, because he has developed a different association. He now associates spiders with the funny things the psychotherapist did during the session, where he was caught by surprise and completely shocked by what happened.

Another American psychotherapist I know would splash cold water on people's faces at the time they were describing their fears or feelings of bad habits. Again, it breaks the association with their habits or phobias.

So the trick is to get eating disorder sufferers to break their association with food by interrupting their thought processes when they feel compelled not to eat, or eat and purge, right?

I was thinking for some time how I could apply this method to Amy. I knew she was a vulnerable girl, so the thought of throwing water on her face would be inappropriate, and jumping around like a clown in front of her did not suit my personality (although I think it's great, and if you can do it, it would be helpful, for sure—it just was not me).

So, I was thinking about what I could invent that would suit my personality to interrupt Amy's food associations.

Once, I went to a seminar by a good hypnotherapist who was talking about breaking behavioral patterns with a totally different approach that was based on fun (cartoon therapy). I thought: This could be what I have been looking for.

Cartoon therapy is when a person learns to associate their own negative feelings with their favorite cartoon music or action.

You can use any cartoon characters, but I used the Flintstones because it was Amy's favorite.

Remember the Flintstones? Wilma and Fred, Pebbles and little Bam Bam. Now what did Bam Bam always do? He would walk around with his club and he would go BAM! BAM! He would crush anything in front of him that he did not like.

How is all this related to eating disorders, you may ask? Let me explain...

Imagine your mind is a computer that plays a program every time you get the urge to starve yourself, or eat and purge. You are simply playing that old program that you made inside your head, all by yourself.

I noticed that Amy had a strong desire to binge and purge, or starve herself when she felt insecure, uptight, stressed, or lonely. When she had any of these feelings, she absolutely had no control over her eating habits.

So she used food (starvation, or binge and purge) as a coping mechanism for the negative feelings she had.

It looks like faulty programming, doesn't it?

So what can you do if you have faulty programming?

You simply get a new one. And it starts by wiping the old program out and building a new, better program in your mind. It is a bit like getting the computer repairman to come around and wipe the old program and install a new one.

I had a recording of The Flintstones music on audio and video. Whenever I noticed Amy looking sad, stressed, on the edge, or withdrawn, I would turn on the music from the Flintstones and tell her, "BAM it, Amy!" "BAM it again and again."

At first Amy looked like, "What's going on?" and did not understand what it was all about. But it was what I needed; to break the cycle you need to do something unexpectedly. I did it a few times more.

It worked exactly the same way as the psychotherapist did when he threw water on the person's face when the person was describing his feelings. Or the other psychotherapist

who jumped from his chair and started making funny movements and shouting "Yam, yam, yam, yam."

Then I taught Amy how to do it when she felt uptight, stressed,
lonely, or just down.

I also taught her how to BAM her negative feelings: sit on a
chair, close your eyes, and acknowledge your feelings (whatever
they are: anxiety, guilt, embarrassment, loneliness, or fear). Then
turn the Flintstones on in your mind, make a fist with your hand,
and say BAM while jumping up from the chair and throwing
your fist up in the air.

What this did was break the negative emotional state Amy
was in.

I also got her to use more empowering words in her self- talk.
When she felt uncomfortable (the time when she would start
thinking about binging, purging, or starving herself for a few
days), she would play the Flintstones in her mind and say BAM
BAM to her own thoughts and feelings, exactly like what little
Bam Bam did with things he did not like.

Later on she learned it so well that she even did it in her
thoughts, without turning the audio or video on and without
saying it aloud.

Now, she can BAM any negative feeling easily.

Of course, it took some time to master this technique, but over
time it worked wonderfully well.

All of the above examples can be called interrupting the negative thought cycle that put you in the stage of binging, purging,
or starving yourself in the first place.

This exercise is better done with someone (a friend, relative, parent, or anyone else who is willing to help).

This someone should also be creative enough to come up with a sudden, unexpected response.

In reality, you can create many ways to interrupt someone's behavioral pattern if you really start thinking about it.

Remember, I told you about the special new programs you can get that affect your limbic system (the part of the brain that we call subconscious)? These programs can change your mental associations with food if you work with them. Also, these programs will help you create a new association with food—a healthy one, like food being a fuel for life, not a mechanism for coping or getting pleasure.

I will tell you about one of these programs later.

PART 9: ELIMINATING LIMITING BELIEFS

The problem with eating disorder sufferers is they have an entire suitcase full of limiting beliefs (emotional blockage) that hold them back and a big reason for the person becoming anorexic or bulimic to start with.

Eating disorder sufferers keep saying things to themselves like: "I have low self-esteem," "I am not capable," "Nothing good ever happens to me," "I feel insecure," "I am sick," "I am tired," and the list goes on.

But our body is really the product of our thoughts. If you continue to say negative stuff about yourself and think negatively about yourself, you will get more negative back. That's why you have an eating disorder.

To cure yourself from an eating disorder you should complete-ly eliminate your limiting beliefs and replace them with healthy and powerful beliefs.

Now, you already know what limiting beliefs you have, as you have done the "Who are you" exercise a number of times (if not, do it).

So now you have to break these beliefs and replace them with positive ones, like: "I feel great," "I am more than capable to manage any problems," "Everything good happens to me," "I have a challenge with an eating disorder to overcome and I will get stronger," and so on.

The problem with limiting beliefs is that other people are the ones who put these in your head, like people who have said bad things about you (like the girl who told Amy, "Told you, you were too fat," when she did not get the part in the play). You have to get them out of your mind.

Think about this. If someone in the past said or did something that placed these limiting beliefs in your mind and you keep rehashing them, then who is being hurt by them? Is the person who said them still hurting after all this time? No! You are the only one still hurting, so why do you want some insignificant person to continue hurting you? It doesn't make any sense.

Also you should understand that all challenges and problems you have in your life, you have for a reason. That reason is to overcome them and become a stronger person, or to start think-ing and doing things in a different way, or to discover something new in your life. There is always a silver lining to any dark cloud; you only have to find it.

This is what you do to get rid of these limiting beliefs:

Sit in a quiet room and relax. Then tell yourself to recall a time when you were really upset, and some other people placed limiting beliefs in your mind. Remember what these people said.

Go back to that time and imagine you are looking through your own eyes. See what you saw, hear what you heard, and feel the same feelings.

Now try to heighten the emotions of the event and as you do, make a fist and imagine you are Bam Bam with his club. Then BAM the bad feelings and beliefs. Don't forget to play the music too.

Now come back to the present. Now tell yourself good things like "I am a strong person," "I feel great," "I have a bright future," "I will win," and so on. Put as much emotion as you can into this play.

Now go back to the past and imagine the same bad scene again, but try and make it worse and heighten the emotions again. Let Bam Bam do his thing again, but try to make it funnier. Imagine Bam Bam chasing these bad feelings around, like in the cartoon, and bashing them with his club; the more action the better. Come to the present and reinforce the positive thoughts again.

What happens here is you replace the old belief patterns with a happy cartoon scene. This breaks the association with the faulty beliefs you had before, which only contributed to your eating disorder. Now it has been replaced by cartoon music and cartoon characters. So every time your subconscious mind tries to go back to those bad feelings, all that is there is Bam Bam.

You should continue to do this with all the negative feelings you have about yourself.

For a more in-depth explanation on the Bam Bam effect see: *Cure your Eating Disorder: 5 Step Program to Change your Brain (The Neuroplasticity Approach)* by Dr. Irina Webster, MD at http://www.eating-disorders-books.com.

PART 10: USING MODERN TECHNOLOGY FOR ANOREXIA AND BULIMIA TREATMENT

For this kind of treatment you will need a simple iPod. Make a recording and load it on to your iPod; a relaxation music MP3 is best.

Play the relaxation music for 2-3 minutes, then have a simple recording device and record your own voice, saying hypnotic and inspiring speech like:

"I love my life because I am happy now and all the time."

"I feel peaceful and relaxed."

"I am extremely happy when I eat three normal size meals every day."

"My food is delicious and nutritious and I enjoy my food very much."

"I am not alone."

"I like to share my meals with my family and friends and they enjoy my company too because we all love and respect each other."

"I think only perfect thoughts."

"I see only perfect things."

"I am a perfect creation of the Universe."

"I am present in the NOW. I am not in the past or in the future anymore. I am in the NOW."

"I am deeply involved in the activities that are happening now and enjoy them."

"I don't think about the past or future, because NOW I am very happy and satisfied."

"I am so grateful for everything that has happened to me. Thank you Universe for my past, present and future."

"Thank you for the challenges and lessons you have sent to me, as they make me stronger and healthier."

"I have ideal feelings, I have ideal looks, I have the ideal body, I have ideal thoughts."

"I am in full harmony with the Universe."

"I am inspired, fulfilled, and happy."

You can tailor the wording of each one according to your needs and beliefs. You may say God instead of the Universe if that is what you believe.

Then, you can play relaxation music again for 2-3 minutes and then your personal affirmations again, then the music for 2-3 minutes. Repeat this several times for as long as you wish.

Listen to these affirmations all the time when you go to bed, go for a walk or a run, wash dishes, or clean your room.

Listening to your personal affirmations and goals in your own relaxed voice will help you change your subconscious mind into the way you want it to be. And if you persuade your subconscious mind to feel happy and have a normal relationship with food, it will be real for you because your subconscious mind dictates how you feel at any given moment.

Think perfect health all the time and these thoughts will make you really healthy.

Dr. Ben Johnson said: "We are now entering the era of energy medicine. Everything in the Universe has a frequency and all you have to do is change a frequency or create an opposite frequency. That's how easy it is to change anything in the world, whether that's disease or emotional issues—or whatever that is. This is huge. This is the biggest thing that we have ever come across."

PART 11: GIVING GRATITUDE

Here is what Amy and I did every morning to perk ourselves up and embrace the day ahead:

We gave gratitude.

We acknowledged all the wonderful things in our life: the gifts we've been blessed with, and the family and friends that fill our lives to the brim with joy.

It's hard to be down and unhappy when you're being grateful.

The point is: Being grateful for what you've got gives you many reasons to be happy.

When you think about it, we're on this planet for such a short time; it's our duty to get out there and enjoy our life. You don't want to look back when you get old and curse yourself for wasting your days in unhappiness because of the eating problems that you did not overcome—but really could have if you had just tried.

You want to look back knowing you gave it your all… that you lived, that you did not waste your talents, that you embraced every minute you had on this earth with grace. So, if you're feeling down, maybe a little bit overwhelmed, then take some quiet time off and give some gratitude.

Write down all the reasons why you should be grateful. Because here's another undeniable truth that took me a while to get: If you're not grateful for the good things you've got now, right this moment, then there's no way you're going to get anymore good stuff. This big old universe doesn't work that way.

It's only when you're grateful for what you've got that you will ever get more good stuff.

What you should do

Every morning, when you wake up, think about what you are grateful for in your life: your family, parents, children, friends, your house, your country, the knowledge you get, the book you have, your health, your happy times, your school, your job, and anything you can imagine you can be grateful for.

If you say, "I have nothing to be grateful for," *that* is why you have nothing to be grateful for—because you've never given gratitude for anything. And once you find the good things that you are grateful for, give gratitude to these. Things will gradually start turning around for you and you will get more good stuff in your life, including good health and feelings.

If you are struggling to think of something, you can be grateful for just anything. Be grateful for the sun in the sky, the nice day that is outside; be grateful for the rain as it waters the flowers. Be grateful simply because you live in the most exciting times.

Be grateful just because you are so unique. So unique, in fact, that there has never been someone like you before and there will never be someone like you ever again. So don't waste the beauty that is you on an eating disorder, rejoice because you are you!

PART 12 (FOR CHILDREN): TALKING ABOUT VALUES AT HOME

This really helped change Amy's way of thinking.

I already mentioned before that I did a lot of reading and learning about eating disorders and their treatment.

In the process, I learned a lot about values in life: about relationships, love, health, and happiness.

I knew that children get a lot of values from their parents, and even just from what their parents talk about at home. Children learn from their parents' relationship with each other and from their parents' attitude to life and health.

I was always hunting for a good topic to talk about at home, so my children could hear us talking and, if they wanted, they could participate. I was really happy if Amy added something to the discussion. And she did from time to time, when she felt at ease.

I did not ask the children to participate in our discussions but made sure that they were around when we were talking.

Parents' discussions influence children's subconscious minds and the way they understand the world.

The topics I chose were:

"Health and beauty"

"Building close relationships"

"Improving self-esteem"

"Internal beauty"

"What does it mean to be happy and how to be happy?"

I really believe that these conversations helped Amy change her mindset and values.

PART 13 (FOR CHILDREN): BREAKING TRIGGER ASSOCIATIONS

One of the main reasons that clinics and hospitals fail is their inability to change the triggers associated with binging, purging, or starving one's self, because most of these triggers are at home, not at the clinic or hospital.

What are these triggers?

They are anything that remind you of your eating problems. They can be the fridge, the cookie jar, a routine you do at home that leads to a binging, purging, or starving episode, or even a person.

To change your associations, you first have to identify them. You can do this by taking notes of what you are doing or have done that puts the idea of purging in your mind; you will find that these are the triggers.

There are many ways to break the associations, but for most, it is not feasible to do some things, like someone splashing a bucket of water on you as you reach for the fridge door, or placing a Jack-in-the-box inside the cookie jar and when you take the lid off, up jumps Jack. These things break the association, but they are a bit difficult to do—so it is back to cartoon therapy.

It is the old Bam Bam principle again, especially if it is a person who sets you off. You have to build a cartoon action movie in your mind around the person and make it so silly that every time you see that person, instead of getting upset, you remember the cartoon about him, and you end up laughing.

If it is your friend or even your relative, if you make them look like Ronald McDonald or Spongebob Squarepants in your mind, you make it so funny that you just can't get upset thinking about them. They may think you have finally flipped out when you are rolling around on the ground laughing, but this is better than the alternative. The same goes for inanimate objects; if you make them look like a cartoon, you can't be upset by them.

To break the association, it is better if something happens unexpectedly, but this is difficult to do unless you are in a session with someone.

It is a bit like the nail biter who uses that icky stuff that tastes real bad on their nails to stop the habit. When the reflex action to bite happens and they taste the icky stuff, they get a big shock. It is not so much the bad taste that changes them; it is the shock. The pleasure is gone, replaced by shock and a bad taste in the mouth—do you see what I mean?

You have to come up with something that you can use on the triggers to change the cycle you have built up, so they lose their power over you. And a cartoon is one that will definitely work.

CHAPTER 4

Mindful Awareness: Relaxation & Meditation

*I*n my opinion, meditation or what we call Mindful Awareness is not just important but necessary for someone who is fighting an eating disorder. It is also extremely useful for caregivers who are helping their loved ones to stop their eating disorder (ED).

Now I expect comments to be raised against meditation, something like:

- I tried meditation and it didn't work for me.

or

- Meditation makes me more nervous because when I meditate my head is thinking about things I have to do and about previous things that happened to me.

or even

- Meditation is a waste of time because you only sit quietly. I need active treatment that involves action, etc.

Yes, I understand all of this because it is exactly what Amy told me before she got the hang of it. It is also what other sufferers have told me before they get the hang of it and learn how to meditate correctly.

I want to be clear at this point? I am not talking about meditation that people automatically think of: the guru sitting on a mountain or a Zen monk. I am talking about Mindful Awareness: the ability to tune into your subconscious mind, feelings and emotions within yourself.

Now I want to answer why some people think negative about doing meditation.

First, if you tried meditation and it didn't work, it was because you couldn't focus or concentrate: a huge problem for ED sufferers at the best of times. People who are stressed and emotionally vulnerable often have problems with the attention system in their brain, which doesn't work properly due to their affliction. The attention system (a certain part inside the brain) can only be put in balance by evoking a relaxation response.

The Relaxation response makes the brain naturally produce certain chemicals in the blood which are used for healing and even curing many diseases.

The relaxation response can only be evoked by doing regular meditation (Mindful Awareness). The more you meditate the stronger your attention system in the brain becomes. Building a strong attention system makes it easier for you to switch your attention from negative thoughts and feelings (ED feelings and thoughts) to more positive thoughts (like fun, joy, friends, studies, interesting job ,etc.)

Secondly, when people say that mediation makes them more nervous because the only thing they do while trying to meditate is to think about something else, it is also related to their weak attention system in the brain and inability to switch off distractive thoughts. The only way to remedy this is to exercise their attention system and improve it by constant persistence. Meditation is one of the best methods for exercising the attention system in the brain.

Thirdly, when people say that meditation is a waste of time because you only sit quietly and don't do any active treatment, it is not true. You already have your eating disorder because of the overactivity of your brain, especially in the areas of food, weight, body image, etc.

To balance your present overactivity you need to calm down and relax your mind, brain, body and soul. It is impossible to beat your disorder by remaining in the same overactive mode that got you to where you are today.

Relaxation Response

Why is a relaxation response necessary for beating an eating disorder?

People with eating disorders live in constant fear: fear of weight, fear of food, fear of inadequacy, fear of intimacy and relationships, fear of shame and guilt, and much more.

These fears were embedded in the person's brain earlier in life and were strongly emotionalized (the person felt very bad about something when the embedding happened).

Strong emotional memories feed eating disorders, continuously overwhelming the sufferer. The person may not even consciously remember what exactly happens when her/his ED started, but subconsciously they always remember the bad feelings that surrounded the event.

Amy doesn't really know what particular episode in life put her on the way to her ED, but she vividly remembers the disgusted feelings she had regarding her body when she was 12-14 years of age. She hated her body. Now, we can only guess about the exact reasons (grandmothers' death, failure to perform at the Christmas extravaganza, bullying at school, etc.)

Fear

Many emotional memories stem from fear. People feel extreme fear and their emotional brain remembers it. Their brain was once put into a "fight-or-flight" mode by fear. Since then "fight-or-flight" feelings continue to persist.

Relaxation response is the opposite of the "fight-or-flight" response. Relaxation response occurs when the body is no longer in perceived danger, and aides the person's autonomic nervous system function to return to normal.

When a person experiences a relaxation response, the person doesn't have any fears, doesn't have any tension, and doesn't have inadequacy or feelings of not being good enough.

The more people are able to experience the relaxation response through Mindful Awareness, the further away they get from their eating disorder fears. Their fears eventually disappear and so does their ED.

It took Amy a while to get used to meditation until she started to feel the relaxation response. At first, she complained about her inability to focus. Also, her so-called friends on the Internet who wanted to keep their EDs said that meditation is bad and doesn't work, further hampering her ability to change.

I had to use all my pervasive power to make her continue with the meditation. I had to really explain to her that her friends who told her this were only covering up the fact that they did not have or did not want to have the ability to stop. And to make them feel better, they wanted to keep her suffering also.

I had to tell Amy over and over that all this Thinspiration stuff was total garbage and a total lie, designed to ease their own feelings of guilt and to cover up their own weaknesses.

I did (and still do) meditation daily myself. I start and finish my day with Mindful Awareness, so does Amy.

I believe that the relaxation response (from Mindful Awareness) was the one that cleared Amy's head of her fears and obsessive thoughts. Without daily meditation we would probably not be as successful as we were in beating Amy's eating disorder once and for all.

Clearing the mind is fundamental to stopping any eating disorders. No exceptions.

MEDITATION FOR PEOPLE WITH EATING DISORDERS

What kind of meditation do people with eating disorders need? There are many kinds of meditation techniques available these days. How to choose which one is the best for a person with an eating disorder?

Are any methods better than the others?

Meditation is a practice of focusing your attention for some time on specific emotional states, mantras (non-religious), breath, intentions, specific focal points, visualization, thoughts, or simply being aware of what is happening at the present moment.

Remember: don't think because we used the word meditation that you have to become a Zen monk or some kind of guru who sits on top of a mountain in India some place.

We are also not talking about some weird religious cult or anything like that. We are talking about scientific techniques proven by modern day science. In fact we like to use the term Mindful Awareness as this is one of the secrets to beating an eating disorder.

To choose the right meditation technique (Mindful Awareness) for an eating disorder sufferer let's look at what kind of meditation are the most common nowadays.

1. **Body-Centered meditation.** This includes yoga, tai chi, pranayama, and gigong. All of them use gentle movement, deep breathing, stretching and being present in your own body.

2. **Heart-Centered meditation.** This includes Buddhist loving-kindness meditation and Christian prayer. These

practices require a focused attention through repetition of phrases that reinforce loving intention and devotion.

3. **Mind-Centered meditation**. This includes Buddhist Insight meditation, Hindu focus on the "Third eye" and other meditations. These are mantra-based meditations and can be learned only from an authorized master who gives a unique mantra for every student.

4. **Spirit-Centered meditation**. This includes communion with God, Source, or Spiritual meditation. One example of this is "Centering Prayer" a technique in which your intention goes beyond the relaxation or health benefit. In this meditation you have surrender to God that is the Source of your Being.

Each meditation system has certain benefits and people with eating disorders can practice any of them if it is what they believe in.

But as previously stated, we recommend a kind of meditation called Mindful Awareness.

People with eating disorders need a special focus on resolving their issues like stopping urges to binge, purge, or starve while meditating. This is important for them because until they learn to ignore, re-label, re-value, and re-focus their thoughts about food, weight and body image issues, they wouldn't be able to focus on anything else. That makes all the above meditation techniques, except Mindful Awareness, difficult for them.

First, if they learn to concentrate by focusing on how to cope with their abnormal food and weight urges, then this is much more helpful to them.

This special meditation can be done in an upright-seated position, either in a chair or cross-legged on a blanket on the floor, even lying down. The spine is straight yet relaxed. Eyes can be closed to better access a relaxed state. Then by listening to specific guidance (on a CD, iPod etc) telling them how to deal with their urges (binging, purging, starving, etc) they can reach their subconscious mind, where the ED lives.

By listening and following the instruction while in meditative (Mindful Awareness) state, they can benefit and over time learn to control the ED voices that keep them locked into their eating disorder.

The benefits from doing this special meditation are:

1. Reduction of stress and anxiety,
2. Decrease of urges to overeat and purge,
3. Improvement of food toleration in anorexics,
4. Improved confidence, calming the mind, clarity of thinking,
5. Improvement in motivations, understanding of happiness and indentifying their purpose in life.

To get significant and life-changing benefits from this kind of meditation, people should start with as little as 5-20 minutes a day, practiced consistently over time.

Generally speaking, meditation (Mindful Awareness) can help enormously to improve mental, physical, and spiritual health of people suffering with eating disorders.

Many people ask what kind of meditation Amy and I used. We used Mindful Awareness Meditation developed and recommended to us by Dr Irina Webster, MD and her husband, William Webster BA. (More on Dr. Irina Webster's involvement in the treatment of eating disorders in the next chapter.)

Now anyone can access their special eating disorder meditation at www.meditation-sensation.com.

I think their meditation is great and exactly what eating disorder sufferers need.

Magical Benefits of Meditation for People with Eating Disorders

Many researchers have proven that people with eating disorders derive a lot of benefits from doing meditation. Eating disorder sufferers have disturbances in autonomic nervous system, problems with impulse control and many emotional problems. All these can be improved with regular meditation.

As mentioned earlier, human beings are made up of three components: physical, mental and emotional. So again: To correct eating disorders all the sides of triangle have to be balanced.

The Mental side represents the knowledge people learn about their condition and how to cope with it. The physical side represents the natural strength of a person's body which we inherit from parents. The Emotional side of the triangle is the one that always becomes unstable in people with eating disorders.

That's why eating disorders sufferers have very bad mood swings, uncontrollable negative thoughts, long-standing bad feelings and painful sensations in different parts of the body that they try to moderate with food (obsessive eating or abstaining from food).

Emotional strengthening is the key to curing many eating disorder problems. Meditation and relaxation techniques are great strategies to do for emotional strengthening in order to become healthy again.

In order to understand about emotional strengthening, you first need to understand a bit about how the brain works. You're probably aware that our brains work across a range of different levels or brain-wave frequencies. While the range is actually continuous, it is divided for convenience into 4 categories—beta, alpha, theta and delta.

As adults, we spend most of our waking time in the beta area. Beta is where we do our logical thinking, rationalising and planning. Stress also occurs in the beta wavelength but on high frequencies beta waves. Eating disorder sufferers spend nearly all their time on high frequencies beta waves where the problem lies.

Alpha, on the other hand, while still an "awake" state, is that relaxed, day-dreamy state that you can go into when you are doing something creative (eg, painting, knitting) or meditation. It's the time when your mind just wanders freely, and when time just seems to fly by.

Alpha-experience represents a relatively stress-free and euphoric state of being. For eating disorder sufferers, the alpha state helps to balance their autonomic nervous system and correct impulse control problems.

Now here's another important piece of the puzzle: besides containing our feelings and emotions, the alpha (sub-conscious) state also contains our "self-beliefs". Our self-beliefs are the sub-conscious views you have of yourself (the real you), they drive our behaviour at a sub-conscious level. They are similar to the programs you have on your computer that makes it run.

So if, for example, you have a self-belief that says, "I am bulimic or I am a binge eater or anorexic," the behavior that results is that you perform compulsive eating, binging, or starving your-self actions. This becomes the real you even if you consciously don't want to become that person.

Where do self-beliefs come from? Mostly they develop in us at a very young age up to when we are teenagers. These self-beliefs go through many developmental stages throughout our lives. It's interesting to note that, unlike adults, children spend the majority of their waking time in the alpha region and this is why they are so resilient.

Most of our adult behaviours are based on "programming" we picked up before the age of 7. Many eating disorder sufferers picked up their programming when they where youngsters to teenagers.

When it comes to getting results, your self-belief (program-ming) will always win out over your conscious desire. So it does not matter if you get up every morning swearing that you will eat today, or you will not binge, but by the end of the day you have not done what you said you would do. This is because you are in the beta state and this cannot affect the subconscious mind, so you are doomed from the start.

That's why it seems impossible for many people to stop their eating disorders. But the problem is that they try to fight it with their logical conscious mind, being in a beta state, not an alpha state.

TARGETING AN EATING DISORDER FROM THE ALPHA STATE

What happens when you target an eating disorder from the alpha state?

Well, you will get a completely different result. Being in alpha state, you will target the emotional core of the eating disorders self-beliefs. When sufferers start to change their self-beliefs, then the magic occurs. Then they can be cured from their eating problems.

Specific meditation that targets people's self-beliefs can create a real magic in the sufferer's life. For eating disorder sufferers who put themselves in an alpha state while meditating regularly, this means they can stop their disorder for good.

If the sufferer is only ever in a beta state this probably means they will have their disorder for the rest of their life, with no escape.

It has been proven that meditation brings enormous relief for the eating disorder sufferer who starts to add meditation into their treatment methods.

Note: Alpha state equals to relaxation response. The only difference is that alpha state is what happens in the brain (the brain frequency); the relaxation response is what happens in the whole body (including muscles, body organs, blood vessels, brain, bones, tendons and skin—everywhere).

For more information on Mindful Awareness, go to http://www.meditation-sensation.com.

CHAPTER 5

The Truth Behind All Eating Disorders

r. Irina Webster, M.D. has contributed quite a bit of input into this book. For those of you who know her, you are probably aware that she is very passionate about eating disorders and helping people to be free from this affliction.

And you may even know that one of the main reasons she is so passionate about eating disorders is she suffered for years from anorexia and bulimia herself.

But what you probably don't know is she has been working on a project for years, and has finally come up with the truth behind all eating disorders.

Dr. Irina wanted me to share with you what she has found, but before I do, I would like to share a little of her own story with you, so you can see why she wants to help as many people as she can.

Dr. Irina always says her story is not as bad as those of others who have developed an eating disorder, but I can tell you that for any child to go through what she did, it could be traumatic.

You see, on school days and on most weekends, she was forced to study for hours after school with no contact outside of the house. Her friends soon learned not to call her, or drop around after school or on the weekends, as they would just be chased away. (We know children need recreation to develop skills and they get this from playing with other children.)

I will let Dr. Irina herself tell you the rest of her story.

DR. IRINA TELLS HER STORY:

"I soon developed bad eating habits as a kind of escape mechanism; it was more like binge eating. (I ate just to make myself feel better, not because I was hungry.) Soon my mother started to tell me I was getting bigger and to stop eating so much. I didn't believe I was getting bigger; it was just that, at 13, I was more developed than most of my peers.

The problem was that I could not stop eating, as it had become the escape I needed to handle my situation. But because of the pressure I was under, I soon worked out that I could eat heaps as long as I purged it out. This simply became a way of life for me and my bulimia was born.

But don't get me wrong, I do not blame my parents. They thought they were doing the best for me by making sure I had the top grades that I needed to get into university, as I had always wanted to be a doctor and help people.

I think my parents were proud of the fact that their daughter was an "A" student; that was considered prestigious in the place I grew up in. I won all the regional schools events, like best science student, best math student, regional champion, etc. While other kids were getting recognition for playing sports, I was tied to my books, virtually 7 days a week.

Did it deprive me of a childhood? Sure it did. But am I angry now? No, I am not, because, in a way, it has given me an insight into how eating disorders can get a hold of you and change you into somebody else.

It was only when I realized through my medical studies that I was doing a lot of harm to myself that I decided to seek help.

I started to approach my lecturers, as I thought they would know exactly what I should do to get rid of my problems. But it soon became apparent to me that the only help they could provide was to send me to counselors.

You see, when you are young and impressionable, you tend to believe people in higher places, like my lecturers. I thought they would know about all things—after all, they were doctors and they were teaching me all about medicine. But they didn't.

I struggled through the normal round of therapists, counselors, and visiting clinics. I did feel better when I was talking to them, but slipped back to my old eating habits when I was at home.

After a while, it also became apparent to me that I was not getting any real help from them either; I decided that the only person who could help me was me.

But back then, deep inside, I thought: If I stopped my bulimia, how would I get through the day and cope with everyday stresses? By this time, the bulimia had become a habit and so addictive; being without it was incomprehensible to me.

Now, I often think how other sufferers must feel. After all, while I was sick, I was being trained as a doctor, so I had a little bit more knowledge on how the body works than the average person, and yet there I was trapped in the terrible affliction. What must others be going through?

You see, I knew nothing about the real implications of emotions or emotional blockages and the role they play in an eating disorder. Sure, I knew that my problem was emotional in nature, but not one of the specialists, counselors, or my lecturers really knew how to remove these feelings. And they knew absolutely nothing about emotional strengthening that I know about now.

I threw myself into all the literature I could find on the subject, and when all I could find in the mainstream was what I had already tried and what had already failed, I looked elsewhere.

It was here that I found real help and soon started to formulate alternative methods for myself, and finally I came up with a system that worked for me and I was finally free from my affliction.

Once I was free from the bulimia I promptly forgot about it. I made myself forget about it. I have often been asked why I did that, and there is a simple answer: 'professional prestige.' It is simply not a good look for a young doctor to have an eating disorder hanging over her head; it doesn't go down well with your peers."

Emotional Blockages

Dr. Irina never stopped learning about eating disorders. Even though her chosen field in medicine centered on women and children's health, she did come across many eating disorder sufferers, and soon became an expert. And luckily for them, she was able to help by offering them something that really works.

So now I have come to tell you what she has found: "The truth behind all eating disorders"—and why I am sharing this with you.

The truth is, "The only way to beat an eating disorder is to use a Neuroplasticity approach." It does not matter how much you as a sufferer or you as a helper to a sufferer want to stop the eating disorder. Unless you can break the mental conditioning and the mental blockages by building new neural pathways in the brain, you will always fail. No exceptions, period.

You see, for any behavior or regular thoughts we have, there are certain brain maps developed and pathways formed. These new brain maps can start to take up a huge amount of space in our brain until they become all powerful.

Eating disorders take up a huge amount of space in the brain because they affect nearly all aspects of the sufferer's life. When it comes to eating disorder treatment, if it does not work on changing the old neuronal pathways, it is not going to work.

What has to happen is for the sufferer to develop new neuronal pathways and build them around the old faulty pathological ones that is their eating disorder.

When you start using these new pathways (the healthy pathways), they become stronger and stronger and they will eventually replace the old pathological ones (these old pathological ones will fade).

When you realize that it is your brain making you do things in a defective way, you will understand that to create behavioral change you only need to make your brain work differently. And you can do that by focusing your attention differently when the eating disorder urge strikes you.

This is basically what we are trying to do with this book, but there is only so much a book can do for you.

You may wish to stop as much as you like, but without the proper methodology, you are wasting your time. You know how this works. You tell yourself: "I am feeling so positive today. This is it. This is the day I turn everything around." And then the first small incident of stress in your day happens, and all your resolution goes out the window.

Why is this? Why does this always happen? It happens because the mental blockages are still there, controlling your every move. It is those little voices that keep telling you: "You can't succeed." These are the same voices Dr. Irina had that told her she could not get through the stresses of the day without her bulimia.

She knew they were there, and still she could not turn them off. If she, a doctor, couldn't, how do you think a person with no training is going to fair? Not very good at all, and the statistics prove this.

Why is it that more than 90% of sufferers who go through the clinics at an average cost of $30,000 per month or sufferers going to group therapy and years of counseling have such an appalling failure rate? It is simply the fact that the eating disorder does not live in the clinic, or the therapy session; it lives with you, when you are at home or by yourself.

As you know by now, my book does require you to have a little willpower; you have to want to give up. Luckily there is an easier way in these modern times.

I was searching for something that can affect the sufferer's limbic system (the subconscious part of the brain) more readily. I was planning to put together a program on the subject.

But since Dr. Irina Webster is an expert in this area and has a great team of specialists to help, I came to a conclusion that her program is really what I was looking for. It is the best that I have found for accessing the subconscious mind.

Because she has "done it herself" and has helped hundreds of other women and men, her material is practical, highly effective and is similar to my teachings, so I know it works.

It is a program that you can play when you start to get over-whelmed, so you have instant support when you need it—a counselor in your pocket, really—and more importantly, a pro-gram that is designed to remove all the subconscious blockages stopping you from getting better. It also comes fully loaded on an MP4 player for your convenience and recorded by her and William, her coach and mentor. Absolutely amazing!

But not only that, I have arranged a special deal for people who have bought my book: a great discount not available any-where else—just to help you.

So now, you will not be on your own during those vital times when you need help; it will be with you 24/7, all you have to do is listen. When their clients apply everything in the pack, they generally stop their eating disorder completely within 13-15 weeks. The program is perfect for sufferers who are on their own.

It is also designed to be used by the whole family and complies with the latest research that states that family involvement is now considered vital in the treatment of eating disorders. Those sufferers who have gone through conventional treatment have twice the recovery rate than sufferers who had no family help.

And that was conventional treatment, not a specifically designed program like this that already has a far superior recovery rate anyway. But again I knew about this aspect for a long time, it is good that research has finally caught up.

So why not check it out at http://www.eatingdisorder-cure.com/mom1.htm

Read this testimonial and you will see why.

"Today I listened to another 2 tracks and they were fantastic. For me personally, I have such a greater understanding of the program when hearing it as opposed to reading. Although I got so much out of the book, when I listened to the program, it makes it so much easier to get going.

Originally, when reading about the dream board, it sounded great but never really got the true meaning of this tool. I didn't realize until Coach William explained in the program how powerful the Bam exercise really is. WOW! I was blown away.

It makes so much sense and I am really looking forward to creating a dream board for myself and will do it with Cole, my son, too. He will love the project. In fact, I have been sharing some of the information with him and he is so receptive. I know it has already been beneficial to him as he is a sensitive, intuitive little guy, and has so much on his mind sometimes.

I'm looking forward to going back to do the relaxation segment. Once again, I'm loving the program and it is really helping. I feel like I am making progress. After the past few dinners, I have talked myself into eating a normal meal and accepting that it was okay to have a snack. I was able to stop myself from getting to that emotional state where I can't control myself.

How interesting it was to hear that only 10% of my mind is the logical part and how true it is that once out of the emotional binge, that part takes over. Boy! It is great to finally realize that these emotional blockages have been holding me back for so long. I have already gotten rid of so many and it feels so good not to have to binge and purge anymore.

Once again, I am going to burst inside and out about how this is going. I know I have a long way to go, but I feel like I've turned the corner on this journey. My emotions are peaking, tears flowing at my good fortune to have found you and Dr. Irina.

How can I ever thank you enough for what you have done for me and, of course, my family?"

Andra, Canada

More testimonials about the program on www.eatingdisorder-cure.com/mom1.htm

WHAT IS NEUROPLASTICITY?

What role does Neuroplasticity play in eating disorder treatment?

The method I used to treat Amy from her eating disorder was based on Neuroplasticity. I didn't know about Neuroplasticity at the time I started to help Amy. I intuitively felt that what I did was the right thing to do. Fortunately, my intuition was right.

Only a bit later, when I met Dr. Irina Webster and we started to talk about things, that I learned about Neuroplasticity.

Dr. Irina Webster said that what I did was Neuroplasticity methods because I actually helped Amy to erase her old negative neuronal (brain cells) pathways in the brain and made her grow new positive neuronal (brain cells) pathways instead.

Researchers are now suggesting that Neuroplasticity is one of the answers in treating eating disorders effectively. They are of the opinion that our own brains, thoughts, and emotions are not rigid or fixed in place. They can be changed in order to treat and even cure eating disorders.

So what is Neuroplasticity? Let's define it. The first part, neuro, is for neurone (which are the nerve cells in the brain) and plasticity means plastic or changeable. Neuroplasticity is the property of the brain that allows the brain to change itself.

These changes occur in four ways:

1. By responding to the world in a certain way
2. By perceiving the world in a certain way
3. By acting in the world in a certain way
4. By thinking and imagining in a certain way

All these activities can change the brain and the way it functions. With "directed Neuroplasticity," scientists and clinicians can pass onto the brain a calculated sequence of input and/or specific patterns of stimulation to make desirable and specific changes in the brain for the better.

For example, under certain kinds of stimulation the brains of eating disorder sufferers can be made to stop focusing on food and weight issues and start focusing on other things. By focusing on other things (called focused attention), the brain develops new connections between neurons and rewires itself. The old neuronal connections (connections responsible for their eating disorder) will became less and less active and eventually completely replace themselves with the new connections. This is how Neuroplasticity works: by deleting old defective neuron connections and developing new healthy ones.

To make it easier to understand, the brain is made up of many chains of neuronal connections. These chains are responsible for producing certain feelings, thoughts and actions that make people do things. And by changing these connections we can change how they feel and act.

Some eating disorder sufferers may say: "Oh well, I've been suffering for so long so I have probably done some damage to my brain that is irreversible." But according to Neuroplasticity principles, the damage done does not matter and it can be fixed.

Even if some parts of the brain are damaged, other parts of the brain can take over the function of the damaged parts—by developing new brain connections (or neuronal pass ways) and re-routing them.

Having worked with eating disorder sufferers extensively, I have noticed that many sufferers are aware that what they are doing in terms of eating and dieting does not make sense, and is even doing harm to the bodies.

But they still continue their erratic behavior because they can't resist the continuous "voices" in their head telling them that they are fat and must continue with their starvation, dieting, or continue to binge and purge.

When you ask them "What do you think the voice is?" They normally answer that it is their brain telling them to do what they do. But when you tell them that it is not their brain, it is their eating disorder (the faulty wiring) telling them to starve themselves or binge and purge. Their thought processes start to change. And when they start focusing on the fact that their eating disorder is something separate from their brain, the changes in their behavior become more profound.

For more on Neuroplasticity, go to http://www.eatingdisorder-institute.com.

CHAPTER 6

Ready? Mapping Out Your Strategies

What we understand from our personal experience coping with a child suffering from an eating disorder is that there isn't one single definitive guide or course of action for you and your child to follow that will guarantee a solution to their eating problems.

Your attitude and beliefs about children and teenagers and their interaction with the parents affect the way you respond to your child.

You should understand that you are not responsible for your child's illness. You should also understand that your child turned to an eating disorder for emotional comfort and is in emotional pain, though she/he may not recognize it.

Remember that if one approach for coping with your child's illness does not work there is always another way.

What I want to say is that people who develop eating disorders are absolutely normal. Something just happens in their lives that make them really suffer emotionally and they turn to an eating disorder to compensate for this emotional discomfort.

SETTING GOALS AND WRITING DOWN YOUR ACTION PLAN

I found it very helpful to write down an action plan on what I want to achieve—and follow it through within a certain time frame. It is better to define long-term and short-term goals.

My first goal was to make Amy admit that she had a problem and needed help. I had to talk to her a few times before she admitted she needed help. You can work on yourself or a loved one to get them to admit the problem exists. In most cases, you know you have a problem and are just hiding it from yourself, to stop feeling pain.

If you are eating less than a church mouse, or going to the bathroom and vomiting after every meal, then you know deep down inside you have a problem. So just admit to yourself that this is not normal, but don't blame yourself or feel bad about yourself. If you fell and broke your arm, would you hate yourself? No, you would seek help. It is that simple with an eating disorder, too.

My second goal was to help Amy take responsibility for her treatment, and help her recognize what personal success is made of and how it feels to achieve and accomplish anything in life. I helped her understand that improvement in recovery, as in life, does not happen through chance, luck, or magic. Things get better because the individual makes the choice and commitment to take purposeful action.

It depends on the situation; you may have other different goals for coping or for treatment strategies.

Using the action plan

Writing an action plan is very important for a successful recovery from an eating disorder.

I used to write and revise my action plan every week. Writing an action plan and setting up goals helped me to subdivide the long process of recovery into small steps and made it easier to follow through.

For example, my first goal was to make Amy admit she had a problem and needed help from us and from outside the family. So I wrote a plan on what I thought I could do personally to achieve it.

I wrote down all possible realistic scenarios for a conversation with Amy to persuade her to admit she had a problem: how and what I would tell her, how I would show my love (hug or kiss her or give her reassurance), among others.

If one approach did not work, I tried another one.

After achieving my first goal (when Amy accepted she needed help), I started to write down goals for the recovery process and what I could do.

I wrote down what books I was going to read to educate myself about eating disorders, and which people I was going to see and talk to about the eating disorder.

Every time I got ideas, I wrote them down. This is how I slowly came to the realization that you have to attack the subconscious mind of an eating disorder sufferer in order to change it back to a normal way of thinking. But not in a negative way. It has to be done with full love and total understanding for the sufferer.

My plans included making Amy accept all the games and relaxation techniques. Some of my goals were:

- Amy should understand and accept the problem.
- She should understand how food imbalances become a bigger picture of imbalances.
- She should learn to name the feelings rather than respond to them behaviorally.
- She should make commitments to restore weight.
- She should make an active choice to let the disease go.

Eventually, Amy started to write down her own plans and follow them through. It is now her habit to set up goals for anything in her life—and achieve them.

This is how Amy slowly recovered from her dangerous health problem.

She has been free from an eating disorder for about two years now. She is a university student studying Child Psychology and wants to help children and adolescents conquer their eating disorders—just as she did. She is going to use the same approach that was used on her to treat other people with similar problems.

I am very proud of Amy and admire her strength and will-power.

I really want Amy's example to inspire and give power to other people to overcome their affliction. The things that are possible for one person are possible for others, too.

If you try to fight the disease by yourself, your action plan may look like this:

1. Admit that I have the eating and emotional problem, and that I want to stop ruining my life with bad behavior. Put it all in writing.

2. First, I want to change my thinking pattern because my thoughts affect my feelings. For this purpose I will:

   • Give gratitude first thing in the morning when I wake up.

   • Do the exercise "Who are you?" for 10 minutes in the morning (or at night), at least three times a week.

   • I will use progressive relaxation techniques every time I feel uptight or stressed and also before the exercise "Who are you?" to put myself in a relaxed emotional state.

   • I will laugh at least an hour every week. I will look for jokes and funny movies, and will communicate with people who make me laugh. I will also try to find a funny side to my disorder to make me feel more relaxed around the subject.

   • I will create new mental associations using the BAM technique or cartoon therapy.

- I will build a dream board and put it on the wall near my bed, so every time I go to bed or wake up, I will see the things I want most in my life.
- I will identify and eliminate limiting beliefs about past situations in my life using cartoon characters.
- I will change my vocabulary and my self-talk.
- I will use power words in my vocabulary and my self-talk all the time.
- I will record my personal affirmations and listen to my own inspiring speech while I do housework, walk, sit in the bus or car, and before going to bed.

3. When I start feeling better I will make sure I eat at least three times a day (breakfast, lunch and dinner).
4. I will consume as many calories as is appropriate for my age, gender, height, and weight.
5. I will check on my correct caloric intake on websites and follow their recommendations exactly.

DEVISING AN EATING PLAN

The food you eat should be delicious, nutritious, and most importantly, should not make you feel sick.

You don't want to put on weight from eating your food, and that is understandable.

I don't want to write an essay about the best diet for eating disorder sufferers, because it really should be a very individual thing.

Your calorie consumption depends on your age, gender, level of fitness and exercise, how much weight loss or gain you've had recently, your general health, and what your goals are.

You can consult your dietitian for an exact diet plan if you wish. But I can give you some general recommendation for a good diet. These recommendations assume that you are average on all criteria: fitness, activity level, weight (not skin and bones and also not overweight), health (you don't have underlying health problems), your age (between 20-40), and you have goals to stay healthy and keep your weight stable.

I am a big supporter of muscle-making meals developed by Jorge Cruise. This diet makes your muscles become firmer, more toned, and stronger. And this factor is very important for eating disorder sufferers because their muscle tissues get destroyed after years of abusing their bodies with bad eating behaviors.

Dr. Irina Webster adjusted this diet and made it suitable for people who are in the recovering stage of their eating disorder.

Description of the diet
For breakfast, lunch and dinner:
Fill half of a 9-inch plate with vegetables and the other half with equal portions of carbohydrates and protein, along with a teaspoon of fat.

If you feel that eating a whole plate will make you sick, don't eat the whole plate at once; leave some for later.

Proteins:
Chicken
Eggs
Fish
Milk
Yogurt
Lean beef
Beans

Carbs:
Whole grains
Cereal
Potatoes
Rice
Bread
Pasta

Fats:
1-2 teaspoon flaxseed oil
Olive oil
Canola or sunflower oil
Butter
Any fruit or vegetable.

This is how you eat to build muscle tone (according to Jorge Cruise):

1.   Eat breakfast within half an hour of rising.
2.   Eat every 3 hours.
3.   Stop eating 2 hours before bed.

It's a recommendation only, but you can adjust it for yourself, like eating more often (but very small amounts), especially in the early recovery process. You can eat as often as every hour, but have small servings.

Also, liquid foods (like soup or puree), do not normally give you these full, sick feelings that make you vomit. So, in the early recovery stage, it's important to eat liquid foods instead of solids. Introduce solid foods in your meals gradually, starting from very small amounts until you feel confident that the solids don't make you feel sick.

Abstain from alcohol, because eating disorder sufferers have low tolerances to alcohol, and even small amounts of alcohol can make you very sick.

FAMOUS PEOPLE WHO HAVE BATTLED EATING DISORDERS:

Paula Abdul, Singer
Justine Bateman, Actor
Karen Carpenter, Singer*
Nadia Comaneci, Gymnast
Susan Dey, Actor
Diana, Princess of Wales
Jane Fonda, Actor/Activist
Zina Garrison, Tennis Player
Tracy Gold, Actor
Heidi Guenther, Ballet Dancer*
Margaux Hemingway, Actor
Christy Henrich, Gymnast*
Daniel Johns, Musician
Kathy Johnson, Gymnast
Gelsey Kirkland, Ballet Dancer
Lucy Lawless, Actor
Gilda Radner, Actor/Comic
Cathy Rigby, Gymnast
Joan Rivers, Comic
Ally Sheedy, Actor

* indicates death resulting from the eating disorder

As you can see, eating disorders take their toll on even very famous and talented people. Who knows, your child could be—or may already be—one of them. Do not let your child (or yourself) waste his or her life because of an eating disorder. Give your child the opportunity to develop their talents and become who they really want and deserve to become.

May the Rest of Your Life, Be the Best of Your Life!

An In-Depth Look Into Neuroplasticity

r. Irina Webster, Director of Eating Disorder Institute, kindly allowed me to publish some of her work where she teaches people about the amazing power of our brain, called Neuroplasticity.

You will enjoy learning about it because Neuroplasticity is not just related to eating disorders. Neuroplasticity is related to our whole life as humans.

Neuroplasticity is about:

- Why we can change our brain
- Why we get sick
- Why we can be cured

It is also about our thoughts, feelings, and emotions. Why some of them make us sick, but others can cure us? Moreover, it is about how to make your brain work with only beneficial ones and ignore the negatives.

UNDERSTANDING NEUROPLASTICITY BETTER

Neuroplasticity is the natural ability of the brain to change its own structure in response to new situations, new behaviors, or changes of the environment. Neuroplastic changes occur in a few different ways: by changing the neuronal connections, by sprouting new nerve endings and even by growing new neurons.

Neuro is for neuron, the nerve cells in our brains. Plastic is for "changeable, malleable, modifiable." Without operations or medications, you can make use of the brain's amazing ability to change and transform your life in the direction you want. This ability can help you stop bad habits, change your feelings and cure many diseases including the most insidious ones like eating disorders.

For the past 400 years this new thinking was inconceivable because mainstream medicine and science believed that brain anatomy was fixed. The conventional knowledge was that after infancy, the brain can't really change itself and was fully developed—only at old age when the brain starts the long process of decline was it believed to change.

This theory of the unchanging brain put people with mental and emotional problems under a lot of limitations. It basically meant that if you had a problem like an eating disorder, you more or less have to suffer for a life of taking drugs and being sick.

This kind of thinking made people believe that real treatments for mental disorders are always biological and involve drugs and that psychological (talk) therapy is not biological and just merely talk, and so would not work.

But now, we have important data from psychoanalytical therapies and neuroscience that shows that when patients come in with their brains in certain states of miswiring (mental states) then after undertaking psychological (neuroplastic) interventions their brains can be rewired without drugs or surgeries. This proves that Neuroplastic therapy is every bit as biological as the use of drugs and even more precise at times because it is targeted.

To prove this fact American psychiatrist Dr. Jeffrey M. Schwartz (UCLA School of Medicine) did some amazing research on his patients who suffered different forms of obsessions and compulsions. His patients went through Neuroplastic treatment called "Four Step Self-Treatment Method."

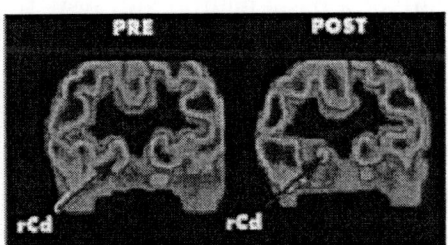

CHANGE IN ENERGY USE AFTER
DRUG-FREE SELF-TREATMENT
WITH DR. SCHWARTZ'S
FOUR-STEP METHOD

Before and after the treatment his patients had a PET scan of their brain. The PET scan showed that after Neuroplastic treatment there was reduced activity in brain's caudate nucleus (the centre of the brain which gets overactive with patients with obsessions).

Obsessions and compulsions are the main components of eating disorders but in relation to food.

So, this research showed that Neuroplastic therapy can biologically change the structure of the brain and help people to be free from their obsessions—without drugs.

To understand how Neuroplastic change occurs read the next article "Structure of Neuron and Neuronal Connections (pathways)".

Structure of Neuron and Neuronal Connections (pathways)

If you really want to understand how the processes of Neuroplasticity occur, you need to start your learning process by looking at the structure of a basic neuron and how they connect to each other. To understand basic principles of Neuroplasticity you need to know that neuron has:

- A body which contain a nucleus
- Many endings – dendrites
- One bigger endings – axon

Structure of Neuron (brain cell)

Axon is a very important structure for a signal transmission. It has a myelin sheath to make the transmission of a signal easier.

The end of axon (axon terminals) connects to the dendrites of other neurons and through this connection signals go from one neuron to another.

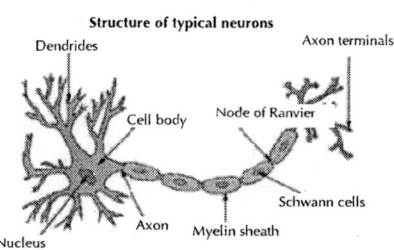

When we think, feel, imagine or dream, all these processes happen because our neurons connect to other neurons in a certain way forming neuronal pathways. Connection between neurons occur in synapses (see picture below) where the axon of one neuron connects to the endings (dendrites) of the other neuron. And the process goes on forming pathways.

So, a neuronal pathway is basically a chain of neurons connected in a certain way. For every behavior, habit, or action we have a certain neuronal pathway. Regular thoughts and feelings also have special neuronal pathways in the brain.

When neurons connect in synapses, the production and release of special chemicals occur.

The structure of synapses (neuron's connection).

These chemical are called neurotransmitters. That's why a signal transmission in the brain is called an electro-chemical transmission. These chemicals (neurotransmitters) play a huge role in our emotions, feelings, and mental states.

Faults in these chemical transmissions can result in different mental-emotional problems including anorexia and bulimia in susceptible individuals.

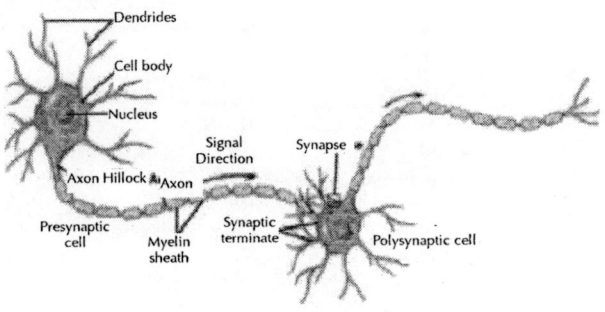

Dr. Ian Frampton, one of the authors and an honorary consultant in pediatric psychology at London's Great Ormond Street hospital, conducted in-depth neuropsychological testing on more than 200 people in the UK, USA and Norway who suffered from anorexia. Dr Frampton and his team found that at least 70% of anorexic patients had suffered damage to their neurotransmitters, which help brain cells communicate with each other.

Luckily, with the help of neuroplasticity, we can now influence even production of new neurotransmitters in our brains around the old defective ones.

Eating disorders are result of "plastic paradox"—when Neuroplasticity goes off track.

Neuroplasticity has the power to produce a more flexible and productive behaviour and even completely change your life from bad to phenomenal success. But Neuroplasticity is not only a good news story. Sometimes it can produce more rigid and inflexible behaviours.

This phenomenon Dr. Norman Doidge calls "the plastic paradox". In his book, The Brain that Changes Itself, he said: "Ironically, some of our most stubborn habits and disorders are products of our plasticity. Once a particular plastic change occurs in the brain and becomes well established, it can prevent other changes from occurring. It is by understanding both the positive and negative effects of plasticity that we can truly understand the extent of human possibilities."

Let's go back in time to when your eating disorder first got started. For instance, your trigger, let's say in the beginning of your ED you were being bullied at school for being slightly overweight or maybe your sport coach told you to lose weight in order to be fit for competition. You were very emotional about these episodes. You were thinking about it all day and night trying to find a solution to lose weight faster. As a result of your emotional thoughts you changed your behavior. You cut down on the amount of food you ate, overexercised, etc. You continued this routine for some time.

And what happened then? As a consequence of your new behavior, you changed your brain; you developed new neuronal pathways that were then responsible for not eating, purging, overexercising and taking laxatives.

When neuronal pathways are developing, they get activated even without your conscious awareness that it is happening. This is why the anorexic or bulimic person continues to starve, binge-purge, and overexercise, take laxatives even though they know they should stop doing it.

There is a saying: "Our life today is truly the product of our thoughts from yesterday." And eating disorders prove this saying to be extremely true. This is because in the past you had a lot of thoughts about dissatisfaction with your weight; today you have an eating disorder.

But the good news is that an eating disorder is not a death or a life sentence. You can stop one by changing the structure of your brain and developing new neuronal pathways which will override the old ones. And Neuroplasticity will help you to do this.

Here is a visual example of how Neuroplasticity works in the brain.

Basic Neuroplastic change (restructure of the brain) occurs approximately in 3 weeks after starting a new regime. Of course, stubborn habits and bad disorders will take longer than 3 weeks to change, especially if they are long-standing ones. Also there are structural brain changes that can occur faster than 3 weeks. Usually these kinds of changes are influenced by extremely strong emotions like fear, anger, or bereavement and can also occur by involving emotional trauma or a nervous breakdown.

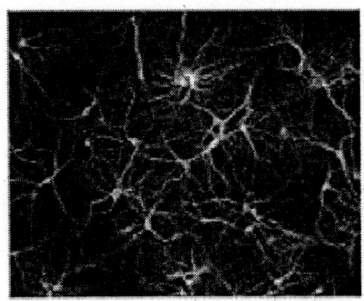

Let's assume that these connections of brain cells is responsible for your episodes of binging, purging or starving yourself. You see how the endings of the neurons are connected to each other.

Then after three weeks of trying to stop the binging-purging episodes using other behaviors (like listening to anice music at the time of binging urges, watching a movie instead of binging, joining a fun club or group, painting or playing piano, doing a course and learning something, etc) .

You see the area in the brain which was responsible for binging-purging behaviour becomes more saturated with brain cell connections. It is because your brain has formed other neuronal connections on the top of the old ones.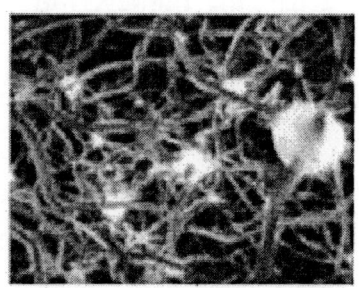

Now, if you continue to perform these new constructive behaviors, the neuronal connections responsible for this behavior will grow more and more, eventually replacing the old negative behaviour pathways.

But if you choose to perform your bad behaviors instead (binging-purging or continue to starve), the old negative pathways take over and the new positive pathways will fade away.

So if you're are serious and really want to beat your ED then it is not impossible, we have developed a book at the Eating Disorders Institute that will help you return to health.

You can get the book online from www.eating-disorders-books.com.

THE 3 MAIN MECHANISMS OF HOW NEUROPLASTIC CHANGES OCCUR IN THE BRAIN?

Biologically it can happen in a few ways:

1. By sprouting new endings from the body of the neuron and connecting them differently to the different neurons.
2. Changing the levels of brain chemicals (neurotransmitters)
3. Growing new neurons (this process is called neurogenesis)

Let's quickly look through them one by one.

1. Sprouting of new neuronal endings will occur when you start doing new behaviors or new actions. These new behaviors have to be done repeatedly and regularly in order to sprout new endings.

For example, when you start regularly performing the act of binging, purging or starving yourself, your brain cells (neurons) sprout new endings forming eating disorder pathways. These are then responsible for the binge, purge, and starving episodes.

You continue because the urge is so strong as you have built these faulty neuronal pathways in your brain.

You may feel that it is impossible for you to stop these abnormal actions but the truth is that you can stop these bad actions by sprouting new neuronal endings and forming new neuronal pathways which can replace the old ones. The mechanism for sprouting these new endings (good one) is exactly the same—you should start performing new constructive behaviors regularly; ones not based on food abuse.

2. Changing the level of brain chemicals (neurotransmitters) can also occur with different behaviors you do. Some certain behaviors we do because the level of brain chemicals remains too high or too low.

For example, neurotransmitter acetylcholine gets produced when people start learning and paying more attention to things they are learning.

Acetylcholine is your attention getter. It gets produced when you pay attention to things and you become more attentive and learn better when you have a sufficient level of acetylcholine being produced. So, memorizing poetry, learning a foreign language, solving math problems, writing an essay, learning about how your brain works, etc—all these activities will improve the level of acetylcholine in your brain.

People with eating disorders often can't concentrate. It is because the level of the brain chemical acetylcholine is too low. But to improve it you must force yourself to focus and concentrate on something useful. Then your concentration will become better because by initially forcing yourself to concentrate you improve the level of this important chemical in your brain.

3. Growing new neurons. Recent research shows growing evidence that the adult human brain creates new neurons, a process known as eurogenesis. Now scientists have found that the areas in the brain where these new neurons grow can be stimulated by actions and neurogenesis occurs. One of the most important areas where neurogenesis occurs is in the hippocampus.

The hippocampus is the middle part of the brain and it forms one part of the limbic system. The hippocampus is directly responsible for memory and our emotions.

People with eating disorders most likely have a chemical imbalance in hippocampus. Eating disorder sufferers store lots of memories of hurts and dissatisfaction with themselves in hippocampus. And their bad emotions come from these memories.

The conclusion is that by growing new neurons in the hippocampus you may help stop your destructive eating disorder behavior.

Now you are probably interested in how you can stimulate the processes of neurogenesis.

Our next article will explain it all.

Tips to Increase Neurogenesis (Growing New Neurons on Top of Old Defective Ones) in Adult Brain in order to stop your Eating Disorder, Anxiety, Depression and Phobias

This is what Neuroplasticity is all about: erase the old messages in the brain and replace them with new ones. The most important thing is to watch what you are trying to erase and what you're trying to embed in the brain. It should always be erasing the negative ones and replacing it with positives ones—not other way around!

Now, let's look at 11 major principles of how we can facilitate the processes of neurogenesis (growing new brain cells) in order to stop your eating disorder.

Neurogenesis is growing new brain cells (neurons).

By now you probably know that eating disorders are problems related to emotions, perception and specific neuronal pathways in your brain, which relate to eating disorder behavior. And that in order to stop your eating disorder you need to create new neuronal pathways responsible for good constructive behavior to replace the faulty neuronal pathways.

1. Learn everything you can about how the brain works. Even some basic understanding will help you to appreciate your brain's beauty as a living and constantly developing structure with billions of neurons and its connections. When you understand what happens in your brain while you binge-purge or starve yourself, you will have an idea of how to reverse it. Until you understand this process you are like a blind person who is trying to find his way home walking through the debris in the wilderness.

2. Take care of your nutrition. Your brain consumes 20% of all the oxygen, nutrients and energy you consume. If you are an anorexic and don't eat (or eat little), your brain starves. It cannot function properly and that's why people with anorexia stop seeing a clear picture of reality that other people see. They see themselves fatter than they are, they judge others by the way they look and how skinny they are. And their starving brain is a big contributor to it. The brain can only function at its best when it has enough energy and nutrition to process the information.

3. Moderate physical exercise enhances neurogenesis (production of brain cells). But eating disorder sufferers have to be careful not to overexercise because many of them already do overexercise. Always remember that when you exercise the spending of energy increases rapidly and body needs energy to burn.

   Energy comes from the food we eat but when there is not enough energy from food, the body starts consuming its own tissue as an energy source.

   Fat burns first. But if a person does not have fat (or has very little) like an eating disorder sufferer, the body starts burning muscles and other body tissues. And that is a dangerous process. It can lead to dystrophy and caxechia—the manifestation of which is a person who looks like he's just come from a concentration camp (we have all seen the pictures). Please remember: moderate exercise is great; I don't mean running 10 miles a day. But you need to make sure that you have something to burn—not just burn your muscles and brain tissue as energy source.

4. Practice positive, future-oriented thoughts, until they become your mindset. Look forward to every new day in a constructive way. Find and follow your main purpose in life.

   Stress and anxiety, no matter whether induced by external events or by your own thoughts, actually kills neurons and prevents the creation of new ones. You can think of chronic stress as the opposite of exercise: it prevents the creation of new neurons.

5. Get excited and thrive on learning and mental challenges. You have probably heard the expression "Use it or lose it."

And yes, it does apply to the brain also. What relation this principle has on eating disorders, you may ask. The answer is: everything.

You see, the brain of an anorexic or bulimic person is full of faulty neuronal pathways which are responsible for their anorexic-bulimic behaviors. There are pathways for binging-purging, for starving, for taking laxatives and diuretics, overexercising etc.

When you start learning new constructive things—like, for example, how your brain works, its anatomy and physiology etc. —you actually will produce new neuronal pathways in your brain which will take the place of your old pathways and replace them.

Learning can be about anything you want to learn but it has to be good, positive and constructive. Something you can share with others and teach them to do the same. The more you learn this new thing the more it becomes your new mindset and the closer you became to eating disorder recovery.

6. Find a purpose. Aim high. As far as we know, humans are the only self-directed organisms on this planet. This means we are the only ones who can make decision and exercise our own will.

    If you don't know what your purpose in life is, don't worry. It will come if you keep focusing on finding it. And don't forget to learn about how your brain works, it also will give understanding on how life has a purpose, which is already created and embedded in your mind.

7. Explore and travel. It has been proven that traveling to new locations forces you to pay more attention to your environment. This will pull your attention away from your eating disorder and help you to develop new neuronal pathways in the brain—different from what the eating disorder has created. It can also help to produce more good chemicals in the brain (neurotransmitters) which are responsible for your attention span. More attention will make your learning of new things easier.

8. Don't succumb to the opinions of others. Don't think that what is in the media, something said by your neighbor or what politicians say are true. Have your own opinion. Remember that media makes billion of dollars every week to program people's mind by displaying women's body images that are impossible to achieve by any normal person. Most diets and other health care products which claim to improve your health don't work or work on a placebo effect only.

9. Develop and maintain stimulating friendships. This is very important for eating disorder sufferers because generally, eating disorder sufferers are withdrawn from others and prefer to spend time alone with their eating disorder.

   By spending your time with good friends, you take yourself away from the eating disorder. You will also develop different neuronal pathways which, if exercised regularly, can replace the eating disorder pathways.

10. Remember: Laughter is the best medicine. Spend more time laughing—it is healing and puts you in a different state of mind. I recommend that you even find jokes about weight and food, laugh at them and look at the funny side of your eating disorder.

    For example, when you see the funny side of being anorexic or bulimic, you will change your attitude from your abnormal behavior. Laughter also improves hormonal status in the body, which normally suffers in anorexic-bulimic people. Laughter also helps to release good chemicals in the brain which can change your brain for the better.

11. Love. Love more, learn about what love is and how you can feel love and be loved. Learn how to give your love to people and receive the love back. I am not just talking about romantic love here. I am talking about love as a number of emotions and experiences related to a sense of strong affection and attachment.

    Eating disorder sufferers don't know exactly what these feelings are—and it is one of the reasons they have their eating disorders. So start educating yourself about this topic and you will discover miracles.

EFFECTS OF EATING DISORDERS ON INTIMATE AND SEXUAL RELATIONSHIPS

Eating disorders affect many areas of a sufferer's life. One of the most affected is the area of relationships (especially intimate and sexual relationships).

The latest research found that people with eating disorders:
- Have insecure attachments to partners
- Have poor quality or absent intimate relationships
- Experienced self-silencing, self-consciousness during sexual activity
- Attempt to change themselves trying to meet the perceived expectations of their partners
- Often have a negative attitude toward their partners and feel that they always attract the wrong person
- Completely avoid intimate relationships and substitute them with their bulimia, anorexia or binge eating
- Believe that if they had to choose between bulimia/anorexia and an intimate partner, they would choose bulimia/anorexia

Why do all these happen?

The answer probably would be that bulimia/ anorexia as a mental state is based on feelings of emotional secrecy, guilt, shame, and anxiety. All these negative feelings override the emotions on which stable intimate relationships are built. It is obvious to everyone that it is impossible to create loving relationships out of guilt and shameful feelings.

Many sufferers treat their partners in the same way they relate to food and eating: unrealistically. They can literally "binge" on their relationships, having numerous partners and being promiscuous for some time but later on "purge" them out by being intolerable, rejecting, blaming everyone and ruining the good relationships they once had.

Refusing to grow up is also an important component of this illness. By changing her body and stopping her menstruation (a condition known as amenorrhea), the woman regresses to childhood and avoids the challenges of normal adults (this includes relationships, sex, having children, and holding a job).

Some patients manage to get married and have children but their relationships don't bring them the proper satisfaction they normally expect from marriage. This can happen for a number of reasons:

- ED sufferers are unhappy with themselves.
- Because of their insecurities and feelings of guilt they may attract a person with psychological problems also (insecure, unstable and addicted to something).
- The addiction to binge and purge can go so far that it becomes unmanageable and their marriage can finish because of it.

Co-existing personality disorders and other mental illnesses also play the role in what bulimics do with their relationships. It is not uncommon when people with bulimia have obsessive-compulsive disorder, depression, anxiety, borderline personality disorder, panic disorders, self-mutilation, alcoholism, drug addiction, and others.

Having co-existing illness is an added complication for them when developing intimate relationships, often making it impossible to begin and/or sustain any relationships. What is a solution for all of this?

Directing the person's attention away from food, weight, body image, and quieting the brain from "useless clatter" is a great first step to helping bulimics overcome their affliction.

Another way is to work with the subconscious mind of the patient, remove the subconscious blockages that caused the eating disorder in the first place. They have to substitute person's bad feelings with positive constructive behaviors.

By doing this, sufferers are able to revive their existing relationships that have turned sour due to their bulimia, or acquire new positive and healthy relationships with the person they like.

Conclusion: First and foremost the sufferer has to take a step back and realise that it is the eating disorder that is destroying their chances of having a full and satisfying relationship.

Being sneaky and secretive about their eating disorder is not conducive to having a successful relationship. Blaming their inadequacies on their partners and looking for the easy way out so they can continue with their erratic behaviour will not help.

The sufferer has to start to consciously identify their feelings and analyse them to see if it is the eating disorder that is talking. If it is, then they have to dismiss these immediately and change these thoughts to better, more positive ones.

Like: instead of thinking about all the negative things about their partner, think of all the good points they have.

The sufferer has to break their conceived pre-programming or the subconscious blockages that are holding them back.

Mindful Awareness has the best result in reprogramming the subconscious mind.

For more information on Mindful Awareness, go to http://www.meditation-sensation.com.

RESOURCES

For anyone who wants to learn more about the treatment methods of Neuroplasticity and Mindful Awareness (the methods that completely cured my daughter from her eating disorder), please visit our websites and you will receive a Special Discount (Karen's Specials) on the recommended retail price.

Karen's Specials

CD

For Eating Disorders Mindful Training CD, visit
http://www.meditation-sensation.com/indexmom.htm

Book

Cure Your Eating Disorder: 5 Steps Program to Cure Your Brain Neuroplasticity Approach By Dr Irina Webster MD, please visit
http://www.anorexia-cure.com/dririnawebster.com/index2.htm
This book will explain to you the much deeper aspects of Neuroplasticity and its effects on eating disorders.

Home Treatment program

A 95-day complete audio program: *Eating Disorder Cure with Neuroplasticity and Mindful Awareness* will help you remove your subconscious blockages which keep your eating disorder in your brain. Please visit http://www.eatingdisorder-cure.com/mom1.htm

For great FREE information and deep learning about eating disorders, Neuroplasticity, and Mindful Awareness, please visit *http://www.EatingDisorder-Institute.com*

BIBLIOGRAPHY

Selective Bibliography and further readings:

Abigail H. Natenshon, *When Your Child Has an Eating Disorder: A Step-By-Step Workbook for Parents and Other Caregivers*, Jossey Bass Inc. 1999

Dr Irina Webster, MD, *Cure Your Eating Disorder: 5 Step Program to Change Your Brain. The neuroplasticity Approach.* 2009

James Lock & Daniel le Grange, *Help Your Teenager Beat an Eating Disorder*, The Guilford Press, 2005

Norman Doidge MD, *The Brain that Changes Itself.* Penguin Books 2007

The Flintstones, Hanna-Barbera Production 1960

ABOUT THE AUTHOR

Karen Phillips is a quiet unassuming person who did extraordinary things when her daughter faced a potential life-threatening situation. Karen likes to believe that what she did (save her daughter from the grips of anorexia-bulimia) was not extraordinary—and that it's something any mother would do faced with the same circumstances.

Karen would be the first person to tell you that she just did what felt right to her at the time. She calls it mother's intuition. Karen did not know until much later that she had in fact used the power of Neuroplasticity, the ability of the brain to change itself using positive emotional input.

For ongoing FREE support from Karen: go to http://www.mom-please-help.com/support.htm.